Rheumatoid Arthritis - Other Perspectives towards a Better Practice

Edited by Reem Hamdy A. Mohammed

Published in London, United Kingdom

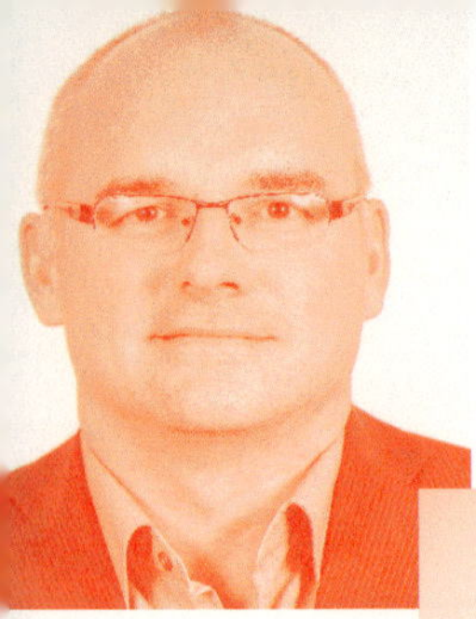
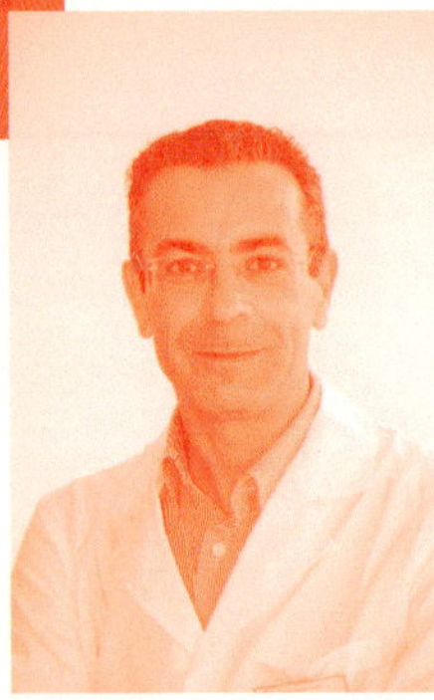
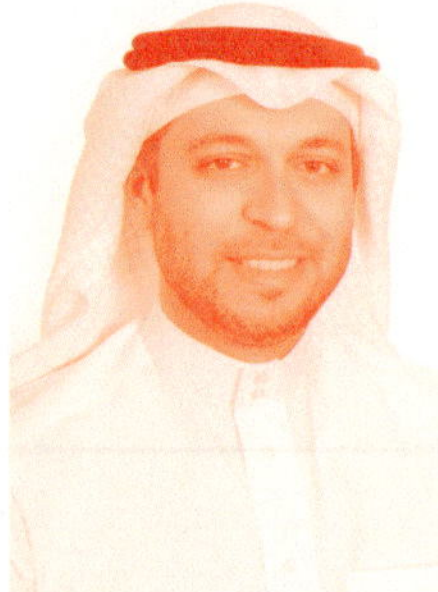
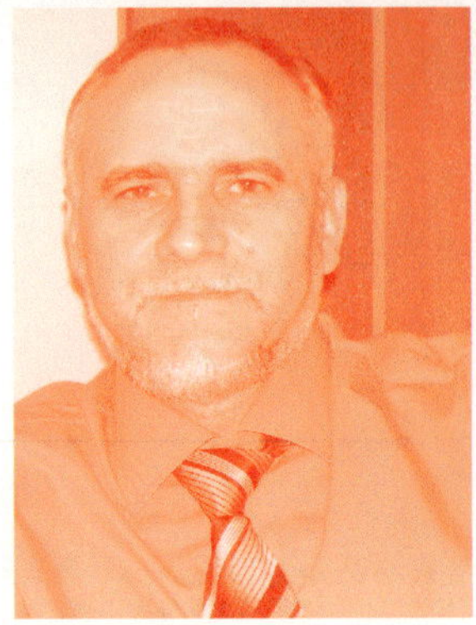
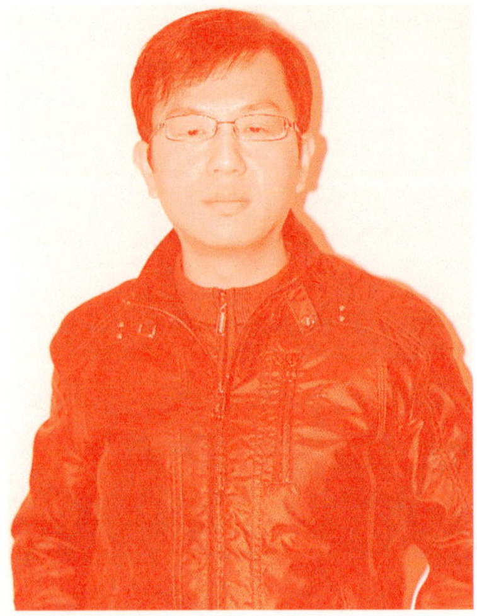
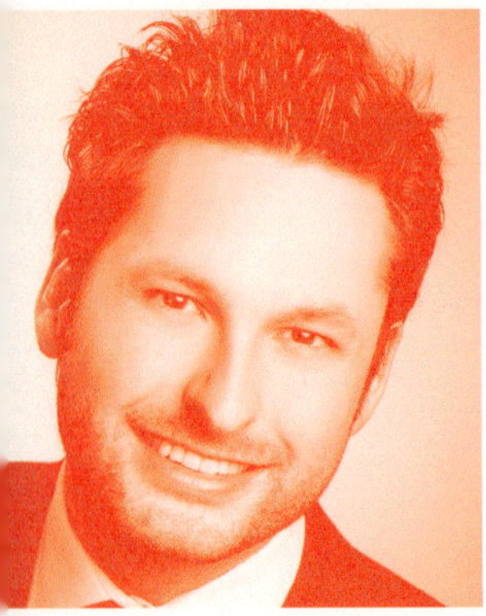
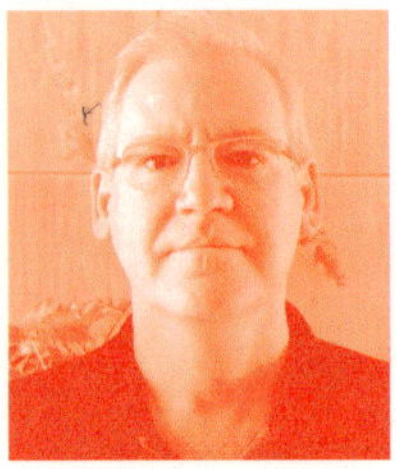

IntechOpen

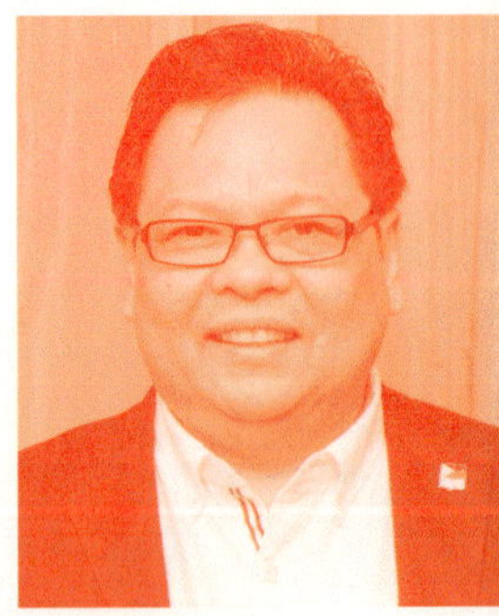
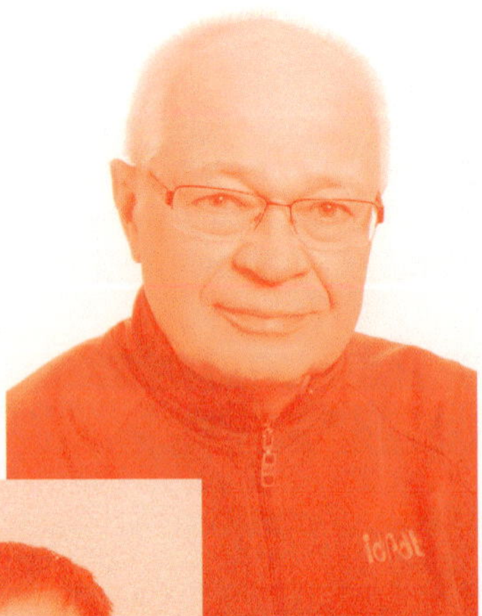
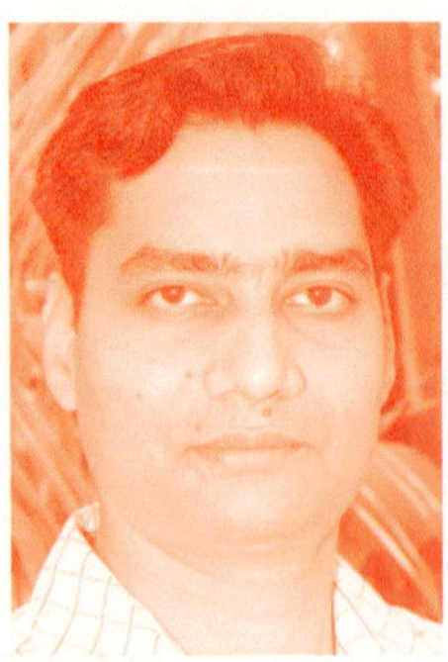
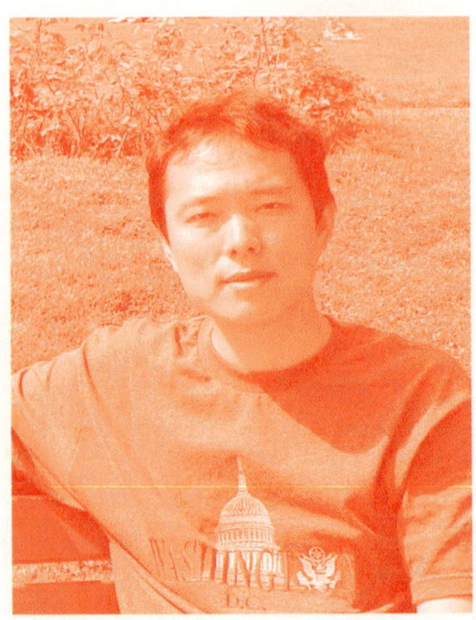
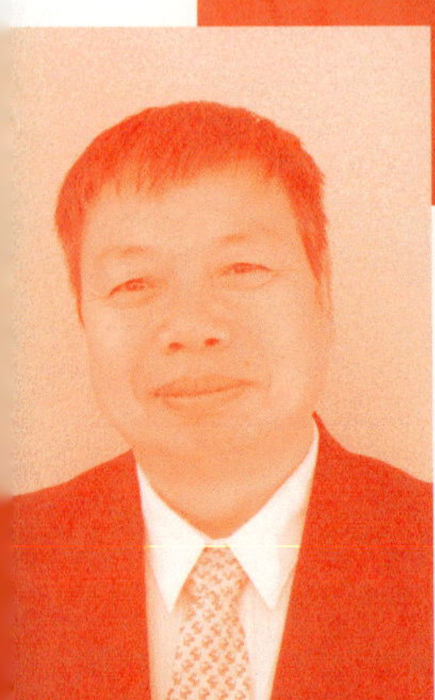
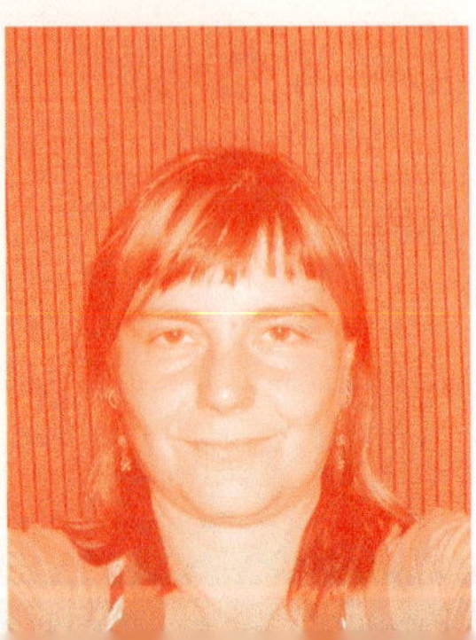

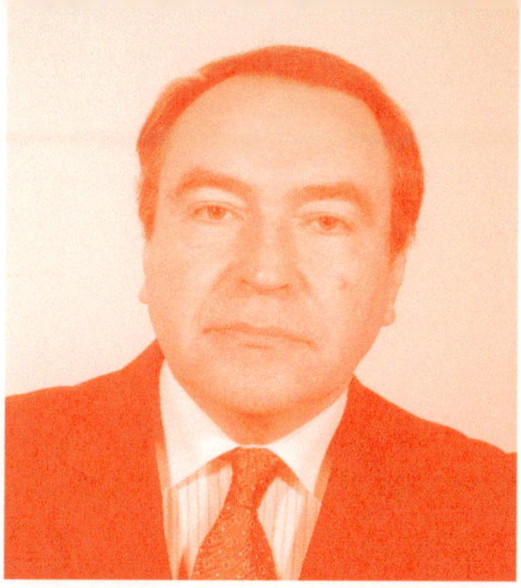
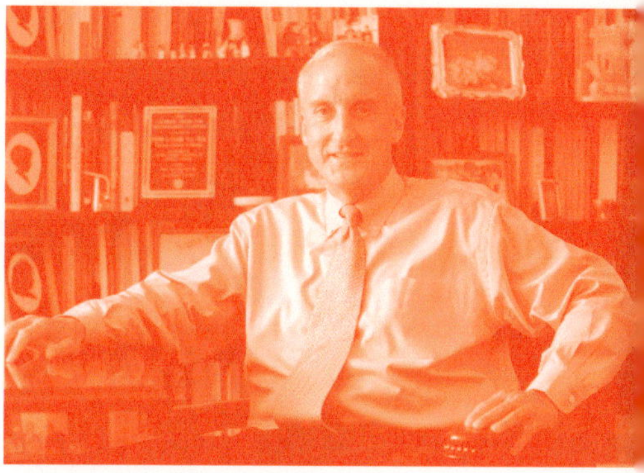
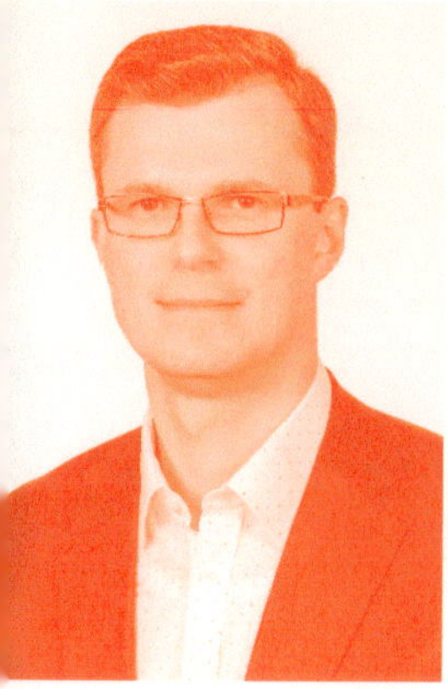
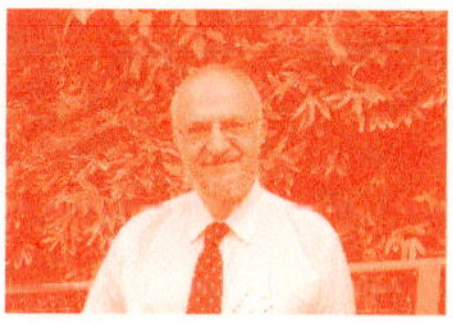
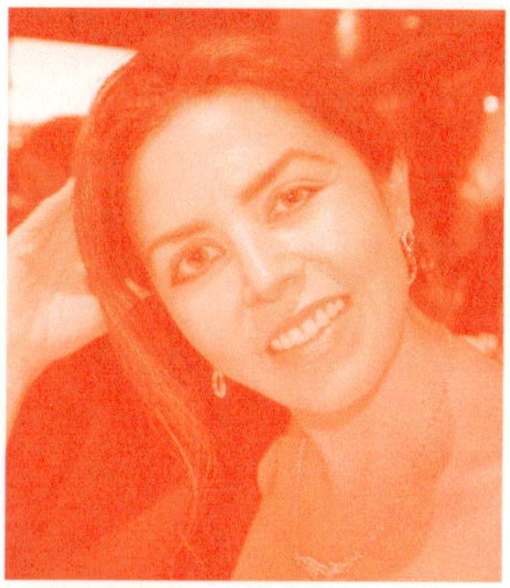

Supporting open minds since 2005

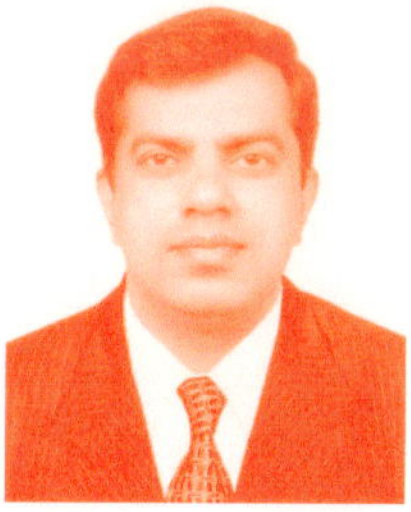
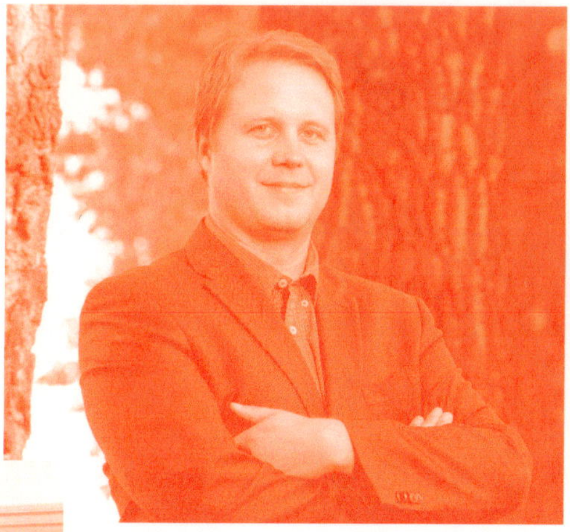
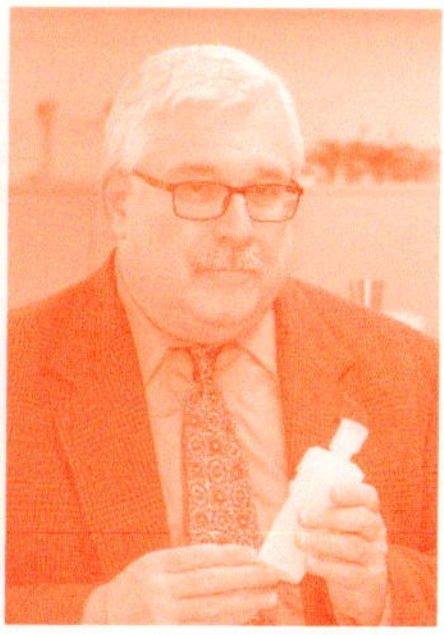
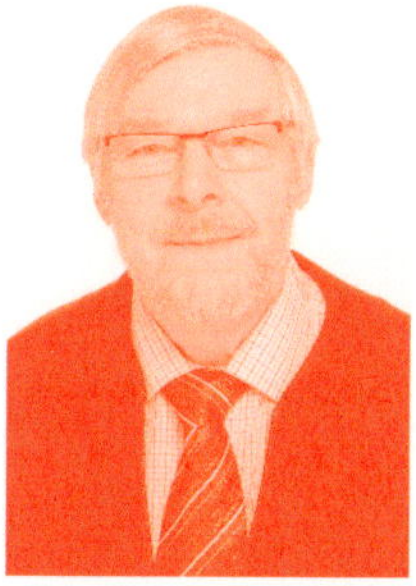
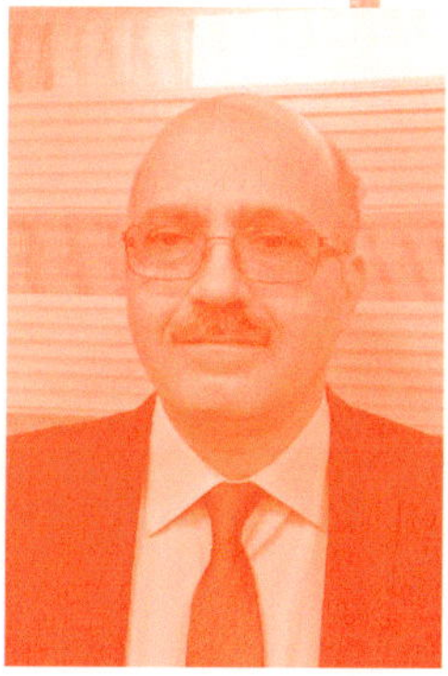
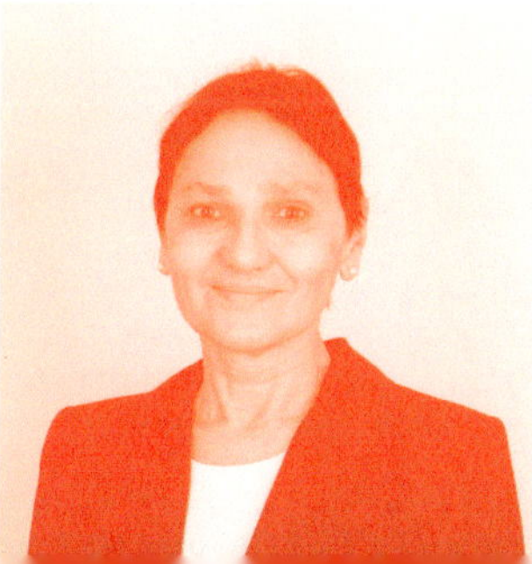
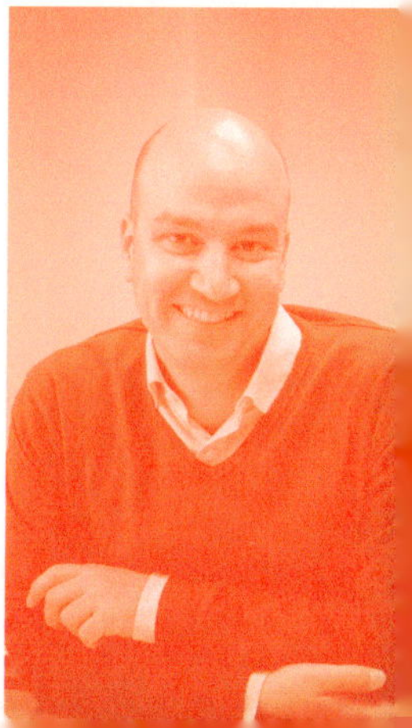

Rheumatoid Arthritis - Other Perspectives towards a Better Practice
http://dx.doi.org/10.5772/intechopen.81489
Edited by Reem Hamdy A. Mohammed

Contributors
Dan Xu, Lei Dai, Jiake Xu, Wen Luo, XiuLi Zhang, Kaijing Ren, Mihail Virgil Boldeanu, Lidia Boldeanu, Florentin Ananu Ananu Vreju, Isabela Siloşi, Bărbulescu Andreea Lili, Andreea Meca, Ştefan Cristian Dinescu, Răzvan Adrian Ionescu, Horaţiu Valeriu Popoviciu, Vlad Padureanu, Rodica Pădureanu, Ioan Sabin Poenariu, Maria Forţofoiu, Mircea Cătălin Forţofoiu, Alexandru Caraba, Stela Iurciuc, Mircea Iurciuc, Julio E Castañeda-Delgado, Maria Fernanda Romo-García, Martín Zapata-Zuñiga, Jose Antonio Enciso, Nidhi Sofat, Kathryn Biddle, Reem Hamdy A. Mohammed

First published in London, United Kingdom, 2020 by IntechOpen
IntechOpen is the global imprint of INTECHOPEN LIMITED, registered in England and Wales, registration number: 11086078, 5 Princes Gate Court, London, SW7 2QJ, United Kingdom
Printed in Croatia

British Library Cataloguing-in-Publication Data
A catalogue record for this book is available from the British Library

Additional hard and PDF copies can be obtained from orders@intechopen.com

Rheumatoid Arthritis - Other Perspectives towards a Better Practice
Edited by Reem Hamdy A. Mohammed
p. cm.
Print ISBN 978-1-83962-532-9
Online ISBN 978-1-83962-533-6
eBook (PDF) ISBN 978-1-83962-534-3

For EU product safety concerns:
IN TECH d.o.o., Prolaz Marije Krucifikse Kozulić 3, 51000 Rijeka, Croatia, info@intechopen.com or visit our website at intechopen.com.

Meet the editor

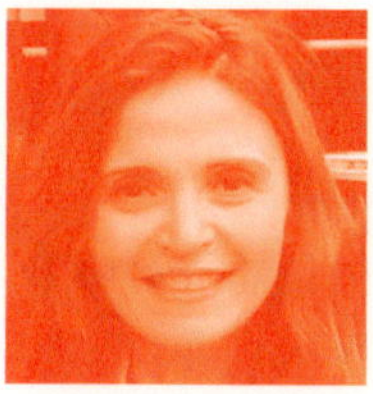

Professor Reem Hamdy A. Mohammed graduated from the School of Medicine, Cairo University, where he serves as a Professor of Rheumatology and Clinical Immunology. She is a fellow of the Royal College of Physicians, an international fellow of the American College of Rheumatology, and a certified international professional trainer (CIPT) at the Faculty Leadership Development Center, Cairo University–Management Development Institute, Missouri State University, where she teaches "Establishment of the Evidence-Based Strategy in Medical Research and Practice." Dr. Mohammed is a verified editor and reviewer for a number of reputable international medical journals. She is the author and co-author of a number of books and an international speaker in the fields of rheumatology and immunology.

Contents

Preface

Rheumatoid arthritis is a chronic, systemic, inflammatory autoimmune disease that typically targets the synovial joints, with a spectrum of extra-articular manifestations. The disease is the most common form of inflammatory arthritis and contributes to considerable disability, morbidity, and mortality. The last two decades experienced an unprecedented leap in the management paradigm of rheumatoid arthritis from treat to relieve, to treat, to target and beyond.

This book examines the disease process of rheumatoid arthritis including information on immune-pathogenic theories, classification criteria, available composite measures of disease assessment, and latest available therapeutic approaches. It also discusses various clinically relevant disease-related problems and comorbidities such as vascular involvement and myopenia. The volume additionally examines the potential benefit of hormones in disease amelioration with a focus on the effect of pregnancy hormones and lactation on the inflammatory process in rheumatoid arthritis. Finally, the book provides updates on pharmaceuticals and patient self-management for better outcomes.

Rheumatoid Arthritis - Other Perspectives towards Better Practice sheds light on different disease-related perspectives that we believe can provide a better understanding of disease-related pathologies and support to improve long-term patient care and minimize related comorbidities.

Reem Hamdy A. Mohammed MD, PhD, FACR, FRCP
Professor,
Professor of Rheumatology and Clinical Immunology,
Department of Rheumatology and Rehabilitation,
Kasr Alaini School of Medicine,
Cairo University,
Egypt

Section 1

Introduction

Chapter 1

Introductory Chapter: Rheumatoid Arthritis - Overview of Current Facts and Strategies

Reem H.A. Mohammed

1. Introduction

Rheumatoid arthritis (RA) is a chronic multi-system inflammatory autoimmune disease of indefinite etiology. The disease primarily affects synovial joints eventually progressing to ongoing inflammation, destruction of both cartilaginous and bony elements of the joint, with resultant pain and disability. The disease additionally displays a spectrum of extra-articular multisystem manifestations [1]. The worldwide prevalence of RA remains underestimated, data gathered from Western regions illustrated prevalence between 0.5 and 1% in white individuals, with prevalence rates ranging between 0.6 and 0.9% in the studied black individuals. The female to male ratio in rheumatoid arthritis is 2:1 to 3:1. A high concordance rate is observed in monozygotic twins 12–15% compared to 2–3% in dizygotic twins [2–4].

Theories behind the evolution of autoimmunity in rheumatoid arthritis are clearly multifactorial. The inflammatory process usually develops in a predisposed individual who is probably exposed to a provocative trigger of autoimmunity via epigenetic modifications. A number of risk factors comprising genetic as well non genetic elements provide the hostile environment for the change towards autoimmunity. Evidences revealed a significant impact of familial genetic risk factors featuring ≥50% of the total risk of developing seropositive RA, with highest incidence rates among first-degree relatives. Among the most influential non genetic risk factors there comes smoking. Smoking provides a stimulus to epigenetic transformation, particularly in individuals with high-risk RA-susceptibility alleles.

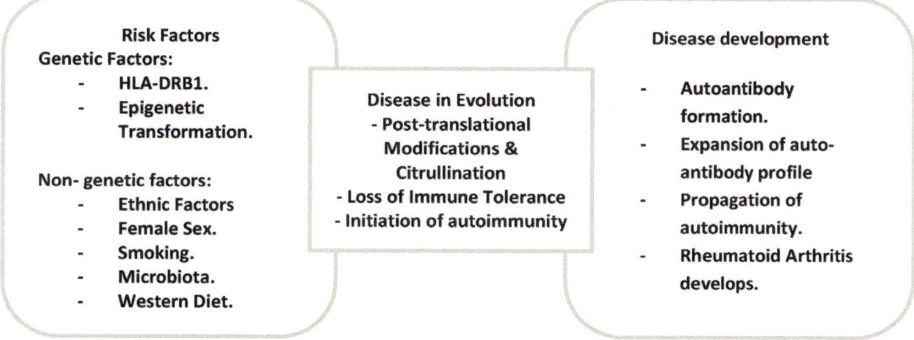

Figure 1.
Etio-pathogenic factors and disease evolution in rheumatoid arthritis.

IntechOpen

Environmental risk factors also include; particulate exposure, periodontal disease, bronchiectasis, diet, obesity and the oral contraceptive impact, respiratory, oral, intestinal and genital tract mucosal sites [1, 5], **Figure 1**.

2. Role players in the initiation and propagation of autoimmunity in rheumatoid arthritis

a. **Neo-epitopes generation**: genetic and environmental factors operate to ultimately result in the inflammatory and destructive synovial response. Stressors including cigarette smoke can act on cells in mucosal sites and promote post-translational conversion of the amino acid arginine to citrulline in a range of proteins, including intracellular proteins (such as histones) and matrix proteins (for example, fibronectin, collagen, fibrinogen, enolase and vimentin) via induction of peptidyl arginine deaminases in a process called citrullination (also known as deimination) rendering them antigenic [6–8].

Citrullination may also be induced by the oral microbiota: *P. gingivalis*, common in periodontal disease which expresses peptidyl arginine deiminases and can induce citrullination. *A. actinomycetemcomitans*, also producing a toxin that increases calcium influx into neutrophils, can lead to citrullination of peptides and has been recently implicated in RA etiology. Post-translational modifications (citrullination, carbamylation, and acetylation) are potentially capable of generating neo-epitopes (neo-peptide antigens). Animal and human data about autoimmunity in rheumatoid arthritis suggest a model in which multiple environmental influences mucosal immune function promoting epigenetic transformations with trafficking of pro-inflammatory PAMPs making use of the enhanced mucosal permeability. Hence, the initial shift towards autoimmunity may present at mucosal sites as reported in previous researches with sputum samples positive for ACPA-IgA and IgG [9, 10].

b. **Major histocompatibility complex binding and peptide presentation**: specific class II human leukocyte antigen (*HLA*; also known as major histocompatibility complex—MHC) loci, which encode MHC molecules *HLA-DRB1*01* and *HLA-DRB1*04* display a very strong association with RA. The altered peptides bind to MHC protein heterodimers on antigen presenting cells, especially those containing the shared epitope [a specific amino acid motif QKRAA commonly encoded by some alleles of the HLA-antigen D-related (DR) locus significantly associated with the risk of developing RA]. Being bound to MHC complex the antigenic epitope gets presented by the antigen-presenting cells (dendritic cells and macrophages) to the antigen-specific T lymphocyte receptor to stimulate T lymphocyte activation and differentiation. Over 100 non-HLA genetic risk factors (loci) including polymorphisms of PTPN22, TRAF1-C5, STAT4, TNFAIP3, and PADI4 have been associated with an increased risk of developing RA [11, 12].

c. **The adaptive immune system**: the activated T lymphocyte stimulates the release of pro-inflammatory cytokines including RANKL, TNF-α, GM-CSF, IL-2, IL-17 and IFN-γ. The antigen-stimulated T lymphocyte then promotes B cell priming via T-B cell receptor signaling pathways then stimulate specific antibody responses by the stimulated B lymphocytes against the neo-epitopes (neo-antigens) promoting a self-directed immune response. In addition to autoantibody production the activated B lymphocytes releases IL-6 [13, 14].

d. **In situ activation of stromal cells**: fibroblast-like synoviocytes FLS, antigen presenting cells and macrophages within the synovial joints gets similarly and synchronously stimulated to release a cascade of pro-inflammatory mediators promoting arthritis with cartilage and bone damage.

FLS masters the intra-articular production of prodigious amounts of MMPs and small-molecule mediators such as MMPs, prostaglandins, leukotrienes, and RANKL. They additionally express IL-6 receptors and specific patterns of microRNAs that could contribute to their activated phenotype. FLS exhibit an invasive phenotype that is responsible for cartilage damage and can potentially migrate from joint to joint to propagate disease. The macrophages like synoviocytes participate actively via local release of TNF-α, IL-1, IL-6, IL-8 and chemokines (CCL19, CCL21) [15–17].

e. **Ectopic germinal centers**: the adaptive immune cells infiltrate the synovial sublining with almost half of the sublining cells CD4+ memory T cells that can either diffusely infiltrate the tissue or, in 15–20% of patients, form ectopic germinal centers in which mature B cells proliferate, differentiate and produce antibodies (rheumatoid factor RF and anti-citrullinated C peptide ACCP) [18, 19].

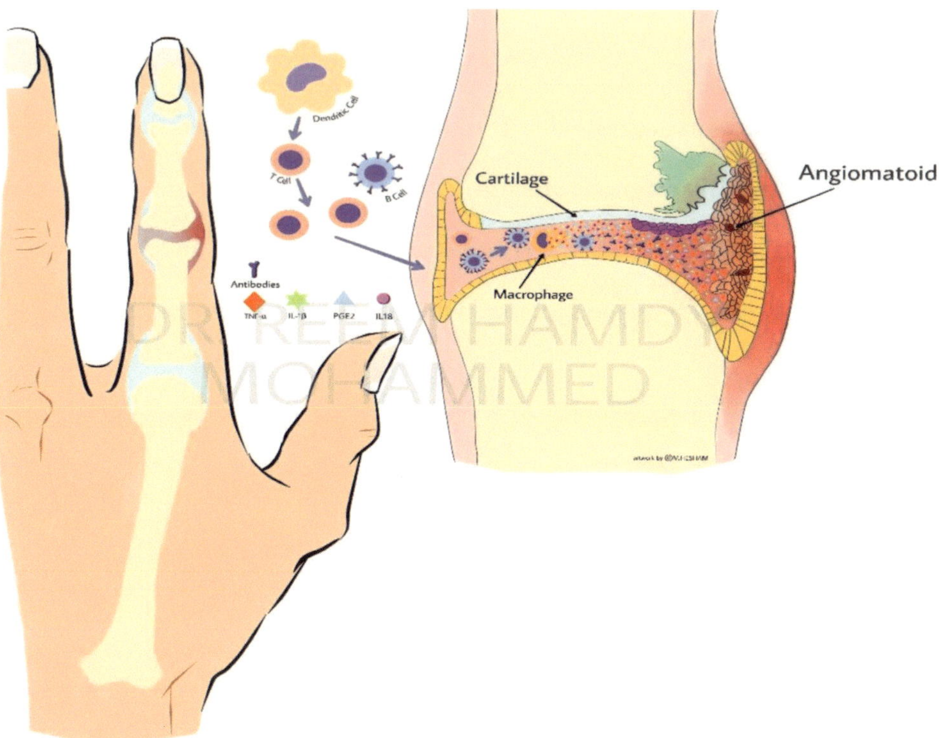

Figure 2.
Proximal interphalangeal joint with macrophages, dendritic cell, T cell, B cells infiltrates with hypertrophied synovium, intra-synovial angiomatoids and pannus formation. "By Dr. Maya H Ibrahim" the original image provider.

The development of manifest disease in rheumatoid susceptible patients usually requires a second hit driven by cross-reactivity, or molecular mimicry to pathogen-specific antigens, in the settings of an inevitable lag of pathogen-immune complex clearance (**Figure 2**).

3. Diagnosis of rheumatoid arthritis

The diagnosis of rheumatoid arthritis requires the integration of proper history taking, careful clinical examination and investigations. Patients might face a period of delay in establishing their diagnosis from weeks to months due to incomplete or intermittent symptoms, defective/unaccomplished clinical/radiographic and laboratory assessments particularly with early disease [20].

4. Patients' journey to diagnosis

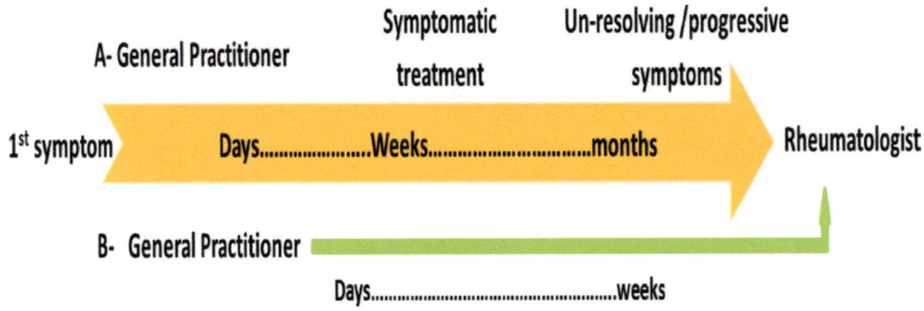

Standard of care in rheumatoid arthritis aims at the following [21]:

- Establishing early diagnosis of RA.
- Identifying arthritis in need of treatment.
- Designing the ideal way to successfully initiate synthetic non biologic DMARDS.
- Providing low remission rates with standard DMARDs.
- Identifying other potential therapeutic targets in aggressive disease.
- Ensuring availability and safety of biologic DMARDS.
- Providing standardized measures for patient assessment, follow-up and treatment modulation.

The recently adopted American College of Rheumatology/European League Against Rheumatism ACR/EULAR classification criteria were established in 2010 with the aim to identify patients with early inflammatory arthritis that is mostly due to rheumatoid arthritis. They have been proposed by the faculty as classification rather than diagnostic criteria to facilitate stratifying patients with similar characteristics for clinical research studies particularly clinical trials with intent to treat. The development of diagnostic criteria for RA as other autoimmune disorders is still challenged by inter/intra-individual variability and chances of misdiagnosis. However, the current criteria might be used to inform diagnostic decision making in clinical practice [22].

5. ACR/EULAR 2010 classification criteria for rheumatoid arthritis

The classification criteria proposed by the American College of Rheumatology/ European League Against Rheumatism (ACR/EULAR) included clinical and serological variables that can be applied only to individuals with ≥1 swollen joint [22].

5.1 Joint involvement and distribution: 0–5 points

Any swollen or tender joint (excluding the distal interphalangeal joints of hands and feet, the first metatarsophalangeal joints and the first carpometacarpal joints) on clinical examination; additional evidence from MRI or ultrasonography may be used to identify additional joints.

1 large joint (shoulder, elbow, hip, knee or ankle): 0 points

2–10 large joints: 1 point

1–3 small joints (the metacarpophalangeal joint, the proximal interphalangeal joint, the second to fifth metatarsophalangeal joints, the interphalangeal joint of the thumb and the wrist): 2 points

4–10 small joints: 3 points

>10 joints (of which ≥1 is a small joint): 5 points

Additional small joints include the temporomandibular joint, sternoclavicular joint, acromio-clavicular joint and others, as reasonably expected in RA.

5.2 Symptom duration: 0–1 points

This variable refers to the patient's self-report on the maximum duration of signs and symptoms of any joint that is clinically involved at the time of assessment.

<6 weeks: 0 points

≥6 weeks: 1 point.

5.3 Serology (according to respective laboratory standards): 0–3 points

Negative for RF (equal or less than upper limit of normal) and negative for ACPA: 0 points

Low-positive for RF (>1–3 times upper limit of normal) or low-positive for ACPA: 2 points

High-positive for RF(>3 times upper limit of normal) or high-positive for ACPA: 3 points.

5.4 Acute-phase reactants (according to local laboratory standards): 0–1 points

Normal CRP (C-reactive protein) and ESR (erythrocyte sedimentation rate) levels: 0 points

Abnormal CRP levels or abnormal ESR: 1 point

A score of ≥6 points is required for classification as definite rheumatoid arthritis (RA).

6. Disease activity scoring in rheumatoid arthritis

Scoring system	Formula	Disease activity states			
		Remission	Low disease activity	Moderate disease activity	High disease activity
SDAI	SJC28 + TJC28 + PGA + EGA + CRP	≤3.3	>3.3–11	>11–26	>26
CDAI	SJC28 + TJC28 + PGA + EGA	≤2.8	>2.8–10	>10–22	>22
DAS	Complex formula including the Ritchie index, SJC44, ESR and GH	≤1.6	>1.6–2.4	>2.4–3.7	>3.7
DAS28	Complex formula including the TJC28, SJC28, ESR (or CRP) and GH	≤2.6	>2.6–3.2	>3.2–5.1	>5.1

CDAI, Clinical Disease Activity Index; CRP, C-reactive protein (in SDAI in mg per dl); DAS, Disease Activity Score; DAS28, DAS using 28-joint counts; EGA, Evaluator Global Assessment (on a 0–10 cm scale); ESR, erythrocyte sedimentation rate; GH, global health (that is, patient global assessment); PGA, patient global assessment (on a 0–10 cm scale); RA, rheumatoid arthritis; SDAI, Simplified Disease Activity Index; SJC, swollen joint count (the number indicates the number of joints taken into account); TJC, tender joint count (the number indicates the number of joints taken into account) [23–25].

7. Different definitions of remission

7.1 American Rheumatism Association

Five or more must be fulfilled for at least two consecutive months—morning stiffness not exceeding 15 minutes—no fatigue—no joint pain (by history)—no joint tenderness or pain on motion—no soft tissue swelling in joints or tendon sheaths—ESR (W) < 30 mm/h (f); <20 mm/h (m) [26].

7.2 DAS/DAS 28 threshold for remission

For the DAS: Ritchie joint index and 44 swollen joint count with either ESR or CRP versions, remission: <1.6

For the DAS28: 28 tender and swollen joint count with either ESR or CRP versions, remission: <2.6 [27].

7.3 SDAI/CDAI remission

SDAI = (28TJC) + (28SJC) + MDGA + PtGA + CRP*

CDAI = (28TJC) + (28SJC) + MDGA + PtGA*

SDAI remission ≤3.3** × CDAI remission ≤2.8** [28, 29].

7.4 Boolean definitions

Depend on meeting a (low) level in each of a series of separate disease activity measures Boolean-based definition at any time point, a patient must satisfy all of the following—Tender Joint Count ≤1—Swollen Joint Count ≤1—CRP ≤1 mg/dL—Patient Global Assessment ≤1 (on a 0–10 scale) [30].

7.5 ACR-EULAR 2011 definition of remission

- For clinical trials: Boolean—SJC, TJS, PtGA, CRP all ≤1 or index-based—SDAI ≤3.3 [30]

- For clinical practice: Boolean—SJC, TJC, PtGA all ≤1 or index-based—CDAI ≤2.8

Factors that contribute to poor prognosis in rheumatoid arthritis include the following [25]:

- Persistently moderate or high disease activity despite conventional synthetic DMARD (csDMARD) therapy according to composite measures including joint counts.
- High acute phase reactant levels.
- High swollen joint count.
- Presence of RF and/or ACPA, especially at high levels.
- Presence of early erosions.
- Failure of two or more csDMARDs.

8. The treat-to-target in rheumatoid arthritis

The treatment paradigm in rheumatoid arthritis has experienced a dramatic shift in the latest two decades. Recently, the strategy changed from a treat to relief to a treat to target. The current approaches in RA are concerned with early aggressive intervention with one or more conventional or traditional synthetic DMARDs (cs/tsDMARDs) and/or biologic DMARDs (bDMARDs) either as mono or combination therapy, in addition to symptomatic anti-inflammatory therapy (NSAIDs, low-dose prednisone). This tight control policy aims to; normalize, sustain or maximize physical functionality via retardation or arrest of joint damage. The treat-to-target is the currently established management approach in the international recommendations provided by ACR, EULAR and the Asia Pacific League of Associations for Rheumatology [31, 32], **Figure 3**.

Recent update on the guidelines of management of rheumatoid arthritis as provided by the EULAR European League Against Rheumatism in 2019 announcing the following overarching principles [33]:

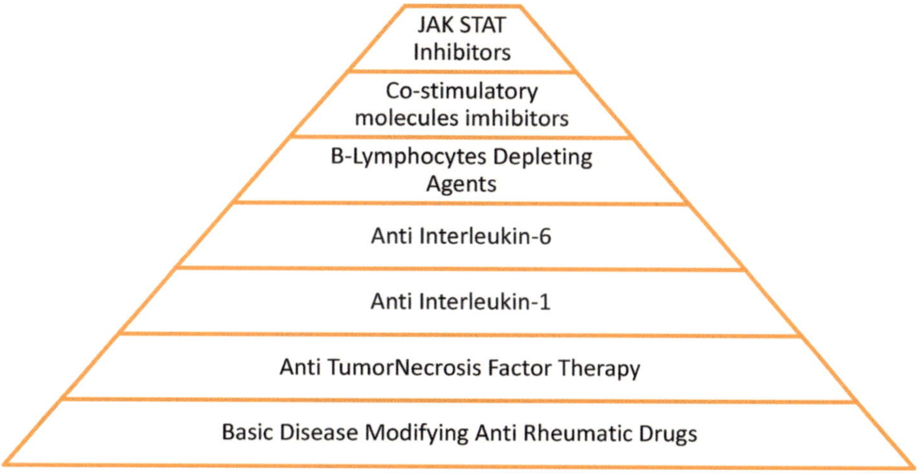

Figure 3.
Identified synthetic and biologic disease modifying anti-rheumatic drugs in rheumatoid arthritis.

- Treatment of patients with RA should target the best care and must be based on a shared decision between the RA patient and the rheumatologist.
- Disease activity, structural damage, patient safety, and other comorbidities, including the risk for thromboembolism must be considered when prescribing treatment.
- Rheumatologists are responsible for the primary care of the patient as they possess the optimal depth and breadth of experience regarding the use of all types of DMARDs, including efficacy, outcomes, risk assessment and knowledge of comorbidities.
- The heterogeneous nature of rheumatoid arthritis mandates patients' access to effective disease modifying anti-rheumatic drugs with successful multiple mechanisms of action.
- RA incurs high individual, medical and societal costs, should be considered while prescribing therapy by the rheumatologist.

8.1 EULAR 2019 recommendations

In 2019 the EULAR taskforce stated a number of updated recommendations emphasizing the strategy to start DMARDs therapy as soon as the diagnosis of RA is made. These recommendations included [33]:

- Treatment should be aimed at reaching a target of sustained remission or low disease activity in every patient. Adopted definitions for disease activity states assessment and therapy include: (a) remission ACR-EULAR remission definition—Boolean or index based, (b) low disease activity state according to any of the validated composite disease activity measures that include joint counts moderate and high disease activity, and (c) respective disease activity state according to any of the validated composite disease activity measures that include joint counts.
- Monitoring should be frequent in active disease (every 1–3 months); if there is no improvement by at most 3 months after the start of treatment or the target has not been reached by 6 months, therapy should be adjusted.
- Methotrexate MTX should be part of the first treatment strategy—the anchor drug.
- In patients with a contraindication to MTX (or early intolerance), leflunomide or sulfasalazine should be considered as part of the (first) treatment strategy.
- Short-term glucocorticoids should be considered when initiating or changing csDMARDs, in different dose regimens and routes of administration, but should be tapered as rapidly as clinically feasible.
- If the treatment target is not achieved with the first csDMARD strategy, in the absence of poor prognostic factors, other csDMARDs should be considered.
- If the treatment target is not achieved with the first csDMARD strategy, when and poor prognostic factors are present, a bDMARD or a tsDMARD should be added.
- Biologic DMARDs and traditional synthetic DMARDs (tsDMARDs) should be combined with a csDMARD; in patients who cannot use csDMARDs as

comedication, IL-6 pathway inhibitors and tsDMARDs may have some advantages compared with other bDMARDs.

- If a bDMARDs or tsDMARDs has failed, treatment with another bDMARD† or a tsDMARD‡ should be considered; if one TNF inhibitor therapy has failed, patients may receive an agent with another mode of action or a second TNF inhibitor.

- If a patient is in persistent remission after having tapered glucocorticoids, one can consider tapering bDMARDs or tsDMARDs, especially if this treatment is combined with a csDMARD.

- If a patient is in persistent remission, tapering the csDMARD could be considered.

9. Summary

- Establish early diagnosis of rheumatoid arthritis.

- Identify patients with arthritis in need for treatment.

- Arrange for evidence-based management.

- Apply aggressive measures to target disease.

- Apply standardized measures for assessment of disease activity, functional assessment, patient and physician global assessment.

- Tailoring of therapy with potential consideration of patient safety, comorbidities and costs.

Author details

Reem H.A. Mohammed
Rheumatology and Clinical Immunology, Department of Rheumatology and Rehabilitation, School of Medicine, Cairo University, Egypt

*Address all correspondence to: rmhamdy@yahoo.com

References

[1] Smolen JS, Aletaha D, McInnes IB. Rheumatoid arthritis. The Lancet. 2016;**388**(10055):2023-2038

[2] Myasoedova E, Crowson CS, Kremers HM, Therneau TM, Gabriel SE. Is the incidence of rheumatoid arthritis rising?: Results from Olmsted County, Minnesota, 1955-2007. Arthritis and Rheumatism. 2010;**62**(6):1576-1582

[3] Tobon GJ, Youinou P, Saraux A. The environment, geo-epidemiology, and autoimmune disease: Rheumatoid arthritis. Journal of Autoimmunity. 2010;**35**(1):10-14

[4] Malemba JJ, Mbuyi-Muamba JM, Mukaya J, Bossuyt X, Verschueren P, Westhovens R. The epidemiology of rheumatoid arthritis in Kinshasa, Democratic Republic of Congo—A population-based study. Rheumatology (Oxford, England). 2012;**51**(9):1644-1647

[5] Malmstrom V, Catrina AI, Klareskog L. The immunopathogenesis of seropositive rheumatoid arthritis: From triggering to targeting. Nature Reviews. Immunology. 2017;**17**(1):60-75

[6] Albano SA, Santana-Sahagun E, Weisman MH. Cigarette smoking and rheumatoid arthritis. Seminars in Arthritis and Rheumatism. 2001;**31**(3):146-159

[7] Harrison BJ, Silman AJ, Wiles NJ, Scott DG, Symmons DP. The association of cigarette smoking with disease outcome in patients with early inflammatory polyarthritis. Arthritis and Rheumatism. 2001;**44**(2):323-330

[8] Hutchinson D, Shepstone L, Moots R, Lear JT, Lynch MP. Heavy cigarette smoking is strongly associated with rheumatoid arthritis (RA), particularly in patients without a family history of RA. Annals of the Rheumatic Diseases. 2001;**60**(3):223-227

[9] Bodkhe R, Balakrishnan B, Taneja V. The role of microbiome in rheumatoid arthritis treatment. Therapeutic Advances in Musculoskeletal Disease. 2019;**11**:1759720X19844632

[10] du Teil Espina M, Gabarrini G, Harmsen HJM, Westra J, van Winkelhoff AJ, van Dijl JM. Talk to your gut: The oral-gut microbiome axis and its immunomodulatory role in the etiology of rheumatoid arthritis. FEMS Microbiology Reviews. 2019;**43**(1):1-18

[11] Citera G, Padulo LA, Fernandez G, Lazaro MA, Rosemffet MG, Maldonado Cocco JA. Influence of HLA-DR alleles on rheumatoid arthritis: Susceptibility and severity in Argentine patients. The Journal of Rheumatology. 2001;**28**(7):1486-1491

[12] Wakitani S, Murata N, Toda Y, Ogawa R, Kaneshige T, Nishimura Y, et al. The relationship between HLA-DRB1 alleles and disease subsets of rheumatoid arthritis in Japanese. British Journal of Rheumatology. 1997;**36**(6):630-636

[13] Firestein GS, McInnes IB. Immunopathogenesis of rheumatoid arthritis. Immunity. 2017;**46**(2):183-196

[14] Klareskog L, Amara K, Malmstrom V. Adaptive immunity in rheumatoid arthritis: Anticitrulline and other antibodies in the pathogenesis of rheumatoid arthritis. Current Opinion in Rheumatology. 2014;**26**(1):72-79

[15] Ferreira RC, Freitag DF, Cutler AJ, Howson JM, Rainbow DB, Smyth DJ, et al. Functional IL6R 358Ala allele impairs classical IL-6 receptor signaling and influences risk of diverse

inflammatory diseases. PLOS Genetics. 2013;**9**(4):e1003444

[16] Firestein GS. Invasive fibroblast-like synoviocytes in rheumatoid arthritis. Passive responders or transformed aggressors? Arthritis and Rheumatism. 1996;**39**(11):1781-1790

[17] Firestein GS, Echeverri F, Yeo M, Zvaifler NJ, Green DR. Somatic mutations in the p53 tumor suppressor gene in rheumatoid arthritis synovium. Proceedings of the National Academy of Sciences of the United States of America. 1997;**94**(20):10895-10900

[18] Firestein GS, Zvaifler NJ. How important are T cells in chronic rheumatoid synovitis?: II. T cell-independent mechanisms from beginning to end. Arthritis and Rheumatism. 2002;**46**(2):298-308

[19] Firestein GS. Evolving concepts of rheumatoid arthritis. Nature. 2003;**423**(6937):356-361

[20] Villeneuve E, Nam JL, Bell MJ, Deighton CM, Felson DT, Hazes JM, et al. A systematic literature review of strategies promoting early referral and reducing delays in the diagnosis and management of inflammatory arthritis. Annals of the Rheumatic Diseases. 2013;**72**(1):13-22

[21] Smolen JS, Landewe R, Breedveld FC, Dougados M, Emery P, Gaujoux-Viala C, et al. EULAR recommendations for the management of rheumatoid arthritis with synthetic and biological disease-modifying antirheumatic drugs. Annals of the Rheumatic Diseases. 2010;**69**(6):964-975

[22] Aletaha D, Neogi T, Silman AJ, Funovits J, Felson DT, Bingham CO III, et al. 2010 rheumatoid arthritis classification criteria: An American College of Rheumatology/European League Against Rheumatism collaborative initiative. Annals of the Rheumatic Diseases. 2010;**69**(9):1580-1588

[23] Schoels M, Alasti F, Smolen JS, Aletaha D. Evaluation of newly proposed remission cut-points for disease activity score in 28 joints (DAS28) in rheumatoid arthritis patients upon IL-6 pathway inhibition. Arthritis Research & Therapy. 2017;**19**(1):155

[24] Studenic P, Smolen JS, Aletaha D. Near misses of ACR/EULAR criteria for remission: Effects of patient global assessment in Boolean and index-based definitions. Annals of the Rheumatic Diseases. 2012;**71**(10):1702-1705

[25] Aletaha D, Martinez-Avila J, Kvien TK, Smolen JS. Definition of treatment response in rheumatoid arthritis based on the simplified and the clinical disease activity index. Annals of the Rheumatic Diseases. 2012;**71**(7):1190-1196

[26] Pinals RS, Masi AT, Larsen RA. Preliminary criteria for clinical remission in rheumatoid arthritis. Arthritis and Rheumatism. 1981;**24**(10):1308-1315

[27] Fransen J, Creemers MC, Van Riel PL. Remission in rheumatoid arthritis: Agreement of the Disease Activity Score (DAS28) with the ARA preliminary remission criteria. Rheumatology (Oxford, England). 2004;**43**(10):1252-1255

[28] Smolen JS, Breedveld FC, Schiff MH, Kalden JR, Emery P, Eberl G, et al. A simplified disease activity index for rheumatoid arthritis for use in clinical practice. Rheumatology (Oxford, England). 2003;**42**(2):244-257

[29] Aletaha D, Ward MM, Machold KP, Nell VP, Stamm T, Smolen JS. Remission

and active disease in rheumatoid arthritis: Defining criteria for disease activity states. Arthritis and Rheumatism. 2005;**52**(9):2625-2636

[30] Aletaha D, Alasti F, Smolen JS. Rheumatoid arthritis near remission: Clinical rather than laboratory inflammation is associated with radiographic progression. Annals of the Rheumatic Diseases. 2011;**70**(11):1975-1980

[31] Singh JA, Saag KG, Bridges SL Jr, Akl EA, Bannuru RR, Sullivan MC, et al. 2015 American College of Rheumatology Guideline for the treatment of rheumatoid arthritis. Arthritis Care & Research (Hoboken). 2016;**68**(1):1-25

[32] Lau CS, Chia F, Harrison A, Hsieh TY, Jain R, Jung SM, et al. APLAR rheumatoid arthritis treatment recommendations. International Journal of Rheumatic Diseases. 2015;**18**(7):685-713

[33] Smolen JS, Landewe RBM, Bijlsma JWJ, Burmester GR, Dougados M, Kerschbaumer A, et al. EULAR recommendations for the management of rheumatoid arthritis with synthetic and biological disease-modifying antirheumatic drugs: 2019 update. Annals of the Rheumatic Diseases. June 2020;**79**(6):685-699. DOI: 10.1136/annrheumdis-2019-216655. [Epub 2020 Jan 22]

Section 2

Pathophysiologic Challenges in Rheumatoid Arthritis

Chapter 2

The Role of Estrogens in Rheumatoid Arthritis Physiopathology

Maria Fernanda Romo-García, Martín Zapata-Zuñiga, José Antonio Enciso-Moreno and Julio Enrique Castañeda-Delgado

Abstract

Rheumatoid arthritis (RA) is a chronic, inflammatory joint disease that can lead to irreversible disability. It affects women in a higher proportion than men (3:1 cases). Several reports suggest a link between female sexual hormones (estrogens) and RA features. It's been described that biological processes where basal estrogen levels are altered like in menstruation, pregnancy, and menopause modifies RA onset, flare, disease severity, and inflammation. Estrogens have a direct action upon the immune system though ERα and ERβ receptors, which have distinct affinity to estrogen concentrations and modifications and have effects upon RA in a dose and receptor dependent manner. The studies focused on dose dependent response at experimental settings reveal a wide (from 25 pg/L to several μg/L) and even contradictory spectrum of effects in patients and cells. This chapter summarizes the contributions and effects of estrogens in RA physiopathology, clinical features, and discusses the possible contributions of estrogen administration and concentration of hormone replacement therapy (HRT) to improve the quality of life and reduce the symptoms of RA patients based on the knowledge of the biology of these hormones.

Keywords: rheumatoid arthritis, physiopathology, immune function, estrogen

1. The RA-gender-hormones link

Rheumatoid arthritis (RA) is defined as a chronic, inflammatory joint disease that without effective and timely treatment can lead to irreversible disability by cumulative joint damage. This autoimmune disease is characterized in most cases by autoantibodies against immunoglobulin G (RF) and citrullinated proteins (ACPAs) [1–3]. The alterations in the immune response is only one face of the disease since it has been described as a heterogeneous disease [4, 5]. This is supported by the wide variation in responsiveness to different rheumatic treatments [6]. Research suggests this might be due to variations in the distribution/expression of estrogen receptors (ERs) in immune cells; ERs often bind to promoter regions in the DNA associated with transcription factors (e.g., NF-κB, SP1, AP-1, C/EBPb) that are important for immune cell function [7].

Phase	Sub phase	Estrogen concentration [E2] pg/ml
Ovulation	Early follicular	30–100 pg/ml
	Late follicular	100–400 pg/ml
	Luteal Phase	60–150 pg/ml
Pregnancy	1 semester	188–2497 pg/ml
	2 semester	1278–7197 pg/ml
	3 Semester	6137–3460 pg/ml
Postpartum	Lactation	35.9–54.4 pg/ml
	No lactation	97.10 pg/ml
Weaning		81.6 pg/ml

Table 1.
Average levels of estrogens on distinct phases of the reproductive cycle.

The relation of immune response and estrogens in RA began with the observation of S. Hench in 1938, where he found pregnancy ameliorated RA, this was the basis for the formulation of his hypothesis sustaining that hormone deficiency could lead to the development of RA, but at that moment, he hypothesized adrenal insufficiency as the responsible of RA pathogenesis [8]. Furthermore, administration of corticosteroids was prescribed for RA patients and the results of the therapy were considered "a miracle cure for RA," but in the case of women, the regulation of adrenal glands seems to be only a part of the therapy. Other studies demonstrate that sexual hormones seem to have a very important role in RA pathogenesis. For example, in vitro studies demonstrated that the achieved concentrations of cortisol do not affect inflammatory cell function, as did the serum of pregnant women, which is rich in sexual hormones. Also the corticosteroid levels return to normality 3 days after delivery, which does not coincide with the pattern of rheumatoid arthritis relapse, common after the third month of delivery [9]. This antecedent opened a new field of study focused on hormones and RA. When concentrations of hormones were analyzed in synovial fluid, a correlation was found in this tissue including, dehydroepiandrosterone (DHEA) which levels are inversely correlated with disease severity and associated with autoimmunity [10, 11] and corticotrophin-releasing hormone (CRH) which levels remain constant in synovial fluids and tissues from RA patients despite the steroid treatment [12]. The dysregulated production of estrogen levels in RA is not exclusive of women; higher estradiol (E2) concentrations and decreased androgen levels have been found in women and men synovia [13]. These concentrations are correlated with those measured in serum in 66% of the patients (14 of 21 patients). The estradiol mean concentrations was 38.25–9.74 pg/ml in serum and 18.83–5.70 pg/ml in synovia; these concentrations showed a positive correlation ($R = 0.79$, $P < 0.0003$) [13–15].

Fluctuations in estrogen levels appear to remarkably impact immunologic profile. Estrogen concentration during lactation is slightly low compared to normal levels (35.9–54.4 pg/ml vs. 63.3–216 pg/ml) upon the normal higher levels (100–400 pg/ml in the late follicular stage) (**Table 1**); together, prolactin and estrogen levels could lead to a change in immune response [16, 17].

2. Prevalence, incidence, and severity of RA in women

Autoimmune diseases affect approximately 8% of the population, out of this percentage 78% are women [18, 19] and for the specific case of RA, the proportion is 3 to 1 compared to men [20, 21]. Also, RA is much more severe in women compared to men (**Table 2**). For example, in a multiple logistic regression analysis for all point and period remissions, male gender seemed to be a strong predictor of remission; for women, the frequency of remission at 18, 24, and 60 months was 30.4, 32.1, and 30.8%, respectively; meanwhile for men, the remission rate was 41.7, 48.0, and 52.4% [22]. Additionally, in another study from a total of 1709 RA patients, (77% female) women had a longer disease duration ($P < 0.001$) despite the fact that at baseline, women had a lower frequency of anti-CCP positivity ($P = 0.03$) and lower CRP ($P < 0.001$), and at 12 months, men achieved remission more frequently (18% vs. 12%, $P = 0.045$) compared to women [23].

The estrogen dysregulation has been associated with disease severity and acceleration of lumbar facet joint damage in arthritis [25, 26]. Added to this, some disorders of the reproductive system seem to increase the risk to develop RA, for example, physician-diagnosed polycystic ovary syndrome (RR 2.58; 95% CI, 1.06–6.30) and endometriosis (RR 1.72; 95% CI, 0.93–3.18) [27, 28]. Suggesting an important role of sex hormones and menstrual cycle regulation as risk factors associated with autoimmune diseases.

These differences could be attributed to the fact that women respond after immunization with a more exacerbated antibody production and an increase in cell-mediated responses. Thus, female patients show higher CD4+ T-cell counts, higher levels of IgM, and T-helper 1 (Th1) cytokine production [29]. This suggests that differences in immune response could be mediated by the hormonal ratios observed during pregnancy and postpartum in women with RA.

There is an increased risk of RA worsening or new onset of disease especially after the first trimester postpartum (**Table 3**), where several immune and hormonal changes are detected like: elevation of monocyte-related transcripts [30], decrease in corticosteroids, estrogen, progesterone, IL-4, IL-10, and humoral immunity, and increase of TNF-α and IFN-γ [31]. These postpartum flares occur within the first 4 months in most patients with chronic RA [32, 33], even a 62% had more affected joints at postpartum; these results were similar when the analysis was restricted to tender joints only [32]. Aggravation of disease activity (in 6 of 9 patients with RA)

Reference	Year	Features men	Features women	Main findings
BARFOT [22]	2007	DAS28 = 5.09 CRP 27	DAS28 5.37 CRP 18	Women had a much lower remission rate than men, although their disease activity before treatment seemed similar
AIR [23]	2014	DAS28 = 5.6 CRP 32 ERS 34 CCP positives 80.7%	DAS28 5.6 CRP 28 ERS 33 CCP positives 74.7%	At 12 months, men achieved remission more frequently (18% vs. 12%, P = 0.045). In anti-TNF failure, remission rates were higher in men than in women
QUEST RA n = 6400 [24]	2009	DAS28 = 3.8 ESR 23 HAQ = 0.8	DAS28 4.3 ESR 30 HAQ = 1.1	30% of men and 17% of women in QUEST-RA were in DAS28 remission
AIR n = 1709 [23]	2014		Lower frequency of anti-CCP (P = 0.03) Lower CRP (P < 0.001)	Female had longer disease duration At 12 months, men achieved remission more frequently (18% vs. 12%, P = 0.045)

Table 2.
Baseline and remission characteristics of RA in men vs. women: comparison of different clinical characteristics of female RA patients compared to male RA patients and the difference in remission rates documented on various studies.

Reference	Period evaluated after delivery (months)	Percentage/fold increase of RA onset
Oka [35]	<6	9.7%
	6–12	2.7%
Del Junco et al. [36]	N.E.	5 fold
Nelson et al. [37]	<6	9.7%
Iijima et al. [33]	12	0.08%
Silman et al. [38]	3	5 fold onset
Ostensen et al. [34]	3–6	66.6%

Table 3.
Percentage of healthy subjects who presented RA onset after delivery or post-partum.

was detected at 6 and 12 weeks postpartum as a progressive decrease in leucocyte counts and increased CPR, whose levels where normal during pregnancy [34].
In the "Pregnancy induced Amelioration of Rheumatoid Arthritis" (PARA) study, 118 patients were followed up until 26 weeks postpartum and levels of autoantibodies anti-CCP, IgM-RF, IgG-RF, and IgA-RF were measured. The median levels of autoantibodies during pregnancy were stable and declined postpartum. When hemodilution was taken into account, an increase in the levels of antibodies explains the symptom onset as well as the start of symptoms due to inflammatory processes directly related to immunoglobulin actions [8].

These dramatic postpartum changes can explain why there is a three to fivefold increased risk of onset during the first 3 months postpartum, with the highest risk being after a first pregnancy [38], in the cohort of Iijima composed by 2547 patients, and the same results were obtained [33]. The available studies on pregnancies in women with RA suggest that outcomes are worse than in the general population [39].

Such RA onset coincides with hormonal changes in the postpartum period, and only the changes during postpartum contribute to RA. During breastfeeding prolactin [40] by itself increases the antibody production and pro-inflammatory cytokines [41] and after the first pregnancy the risk of RA increases several times [42]. An additional link between sex-hormones and increased risk of RA come from data showing that the administration of drugs for lactation suppression which mainly are high-dose estrogens, increased risk of RA development [26]. Given that several cytokines are regulated by estrogens, so a decrease in this hormone could be responsible for flare and disease onset as it contributes to the activation of the immune system necessary for the delivery [43].

Estrogen seems to orchestrate several key features of the immune response and may be a critical factor in the incidence and severity of the disease in women. Small variations in estrogen concentration can have a very wide range of effects, even some of them could be opposite even when they are provoked by the same molecule.

3. Influence of reproductive cycle hormones and their role in RA immune response

3.1 Arthritis and menstruation

Since 1980, it was noted that young women with rheumatoid arthritis (RA) report an exacerbation of symptoms just before or at the time of menstruation, it could possibly be related to "premenstrual tension syndrome" and alteration in pain perception [44], but in a study where only objective measures of disease activity were measured, a significant cyclical change in finger joint size (FJS) was seen in 4 of 7 patients with RA, with all peaks occurring within 6 days of the start of menstruation [45] while on contrary, the morning stiffness was reduced during the post-ovulatory phase where estrogen and progesterone are high [46], indicating that this worsening of symptoms might be related to variations in hormone levels [47]. Based on this evidence, a relation between low levels of estrogen (at luteal phase) can correspond to enhancement of RA symptoms. Contrary to what occurs on pregnancy, where high estrogen levels seem to have a protective effect. Until now there is no follow up study available to display the effect of cyclical variations in estrogen levels and symptoms severity in RA patients.

3.2 Arthritis and pregnancy

As stated previously, the relationship of RA onset and sex hormones has been widely studied. This phenomena was described first 80 years ago [8] and was noticed that pregnant patients with RA usually go into remission [48] in a 20–40% by the third trimester and 50% had low disease activity [49]. Prospective studies have shown that only 48–66% of women with RA experience improvement in pregnancy, with 20% becoming quiescent by the third trimester and 16% in complete remission (no joints with active disease without therapy) [32, 50].

It has been hypothesized that estradiol might be the principal regulator of immune response during pregnancy, nevertheless other estrogens might be implicated in this immune regulation, as an example we can cite estriol (E3) which is mainly produced during pregnancy [51, 52], and estetrol (E4) is synthesized exclusively by the fetal liver during pregnancy being able to reach the maternal circulation through the placenta [53]; thus, these two estrogens, specifically E4 could have an important role in the immune regulation during pregnancy; nevertheless, there is scarce information about its possible function during pregnancy.

A shift from a Th1/Th17 pro-inflammatory response to a Th2/Treg response has been observed in pregnancy [54, 55]. This could explain the decrease of IL-2 during pregnancy, while soluble TNF receptor, p55 and p75, increases [56]. The role of the immune system in pregnancy is very important. It has been observed that a depletion of immune cells can cause the termination of the pregnancy. Nevertheless, it is not very clear how such changes in T helper cell function could impact the implantation process. It has been suggested that the response could be induced by trophoblastic cells that can secrete IL-6, IL-8, MCP-1, and GRO-α, early in pregnancy [43].

During the first trimester, NK cells, dendritic cells, macrophages, and regulatory T cells (Treg) infiltrate the decidua and accumulate around the trophoblastic cells [57–59]. This regulation of the immune response could be the cause beneath the clinical improvement observed in RA during pregnancy.

3.3 Menopause and arthritis

RA onset is common in the peri-menopausal age, which is not the case with SLE [60] and while hormone replace therapy (HRT) is proposed as therapy for women with RA, OCP and postmenopausal hormones significantly increased the risk of SLE [61]. Also, there is an inverse trend for RA incidence when women reach menopause after 51 years compared to those who reach menopause before 45 years of age. This is consistent with a decline in the production of sex hormones and suggesting that changes in immune regulation due to the availability of estrogen receptors in immune cells and circulating estrogens might also have an effect on RA onset on these late menopausal women [26].

4. Molecular aspects of estrogen effects in immune response

4.1 Regulation by estrogen receptors

ERα (NR3A1) and ERβ (NR3A2) that are encoded by ESR-1 and ESR-2 genes expressed on human chromosomes 6 and 14, respectively [62]. It is estimated that both receptors regulate 40% of the genes in cell line U2OS [63], but despite both are estrogen receptors (ERs), ERα and ERβ microarray analysis had demonstrated that they regulate different genes [7, 64, 65]. The activation of one or other of these ERs has specific effects in distinct, non-overlapping or even antagonist effects determined by factors like distribution, expression, dimerization, splice variant ER isoforms, signaling pathways triggered, physiological stage, and interaction with specific co-activators/−repressors [62]. One example of the distribution of these receptors is given in T lymphocytes, CD4+ cells which have higher ERα levels, B cells have higher ERβ expression than ERα and CD8+ cells have lower expression of both receptors [66], murine splenic DCs express ERα but has negligible ERβ expression and bone marrow-derived and peritoneal macrophages also express ERα and few if any ERβ [67, 68], so given the expression, lower or higher concentrations of estrogens will be needed to activate the receptors with the lowest expression [69].

In general terms, the effect of ERα on the immune system is more prominent than ERβ due to regulating multiple NF-kB pathway members to control cytokine responses. This, given that ERs are ligand-dependent transcription factors that mediate long-range chromatin interactions and form complexes at gene regulatory elements, thus promoting epigenetic changes and transcription [70]. Also, its promotion of strong antigen-specific Th1 cell responses was demonstrated in ERα-deficient mice where E2 effects on Th1 responses were not observed [71], apart from but this receptor is not only delimited to the cells at periphery, its expression seems to have effects in the thymus and spleen since deletion of ERα led to hypoplasia of both organs and contribute to the increased frequency of immature CD4 + CD8+ thymocytes and decreased CD4 + CD8− cells [72].

4.2 Estrogen dose and receptor dependent effects

As mentioned previously, estrogen receptors (ER) are expressed in the immune cells; TaqMan RT-PCR analyses indicate that in CD4 + T-helper cells express higher concentrations of ERα, B cells ERβ, and CD8+ T cells; monocytes express both ERs at lower concentrations [66]; this proportion is important because despite both receptors are present in all PBMCs, the functions elicited by their activation vary depending on the proportion of each receptor on such cells. A wider description of such differential effects is made for several cell types:

T cells: CD4+ T responds to E2 administration at low physiological levels (of 60–100 pg/ml in castrated female mice) increasing antigen specific responses, production of IFNγ and IL2 as well as inducing FoxP3 positive Treg cell differentiation [71, 73–75]. During the reproductive cycle CD4+, T cells increase on preovulatory (late follicular) [76], decrease in the luteal phase (60–150 pg/ml) compared to the early follicular phase (30–100 pg/mL) [77] and increased in the first trimester of pregnancy (8.9%, vs. 4.4% of controls) and 6–8 weeks following delivery [78]. Regarding CD8+ T cells, there is not much evidence, in models of collagen-II induce

RA, CD8+, lymphocytes were significantly diminished in the spleen of the estradiol-treated animals and were suppressed in the thymus [79].

Fibroblast-like synoviocytes: on FLS (**Figure 1**), estrogens induce an increase of MMP invasion of cartilage when these cells were transfected with ERα, thus estrogen levels can influence joint erosion degradation of extracellular matrix [80]. Regarding this antecedent, an increase in hormonal levels at synovia could influence cytokine levels but it is not clear if the effects of estrogen upon certain cytokines like TNF-α, IL-10, and IL-6 are unidirectional or could be an initial trigger of aromatase activity. For example, TNF-α, IL-1, and IL-6 stimulate fibroblast aromatase activity in a dose-dependent manner; the aromatase enzyme complex is involved in the peripheral conversion of androgens (testosterone and androstenedione) to estrogens (estrone and estradiol, respectively) [81].

B cells: concentrations of E2 ranging 75 pg/ml or above activate ERs, leading to an upregulation of CD22, SHP-1, BCL-2, and V-CAM-1. This can alter the survival of immature B cells that would normally be deleted [82]. Also a decrease in transitional B cells and increased marginal zone B cells [83] has been observed. In the presence of estrogen, BAFF increased its expression by 5-fold, but this characteristic was more pronounced in cells isolated from women than in those from man [84]. An overexpression of BAFF in transgenic mice leads to manifestations of autoimmune disease [85], and similar BAFF increase has been reported in the serum of patients with RA, [86] even at early stages of RA and correlates with the titers of IgM rheumatoid factor and anti-cyclic citrullinated peptide autoantibody (R = 0.76 and R = 0.49) [87]. It has been hypothesized that high levels of estrogens during pregnancy could prevent B cell apoptosis and therefore enhance survival of autoreactive cells [88]. Implications of estrogen signaling on auto reactive B cell expansion and autoantibodies production have not been evaluated in the clinical setting.

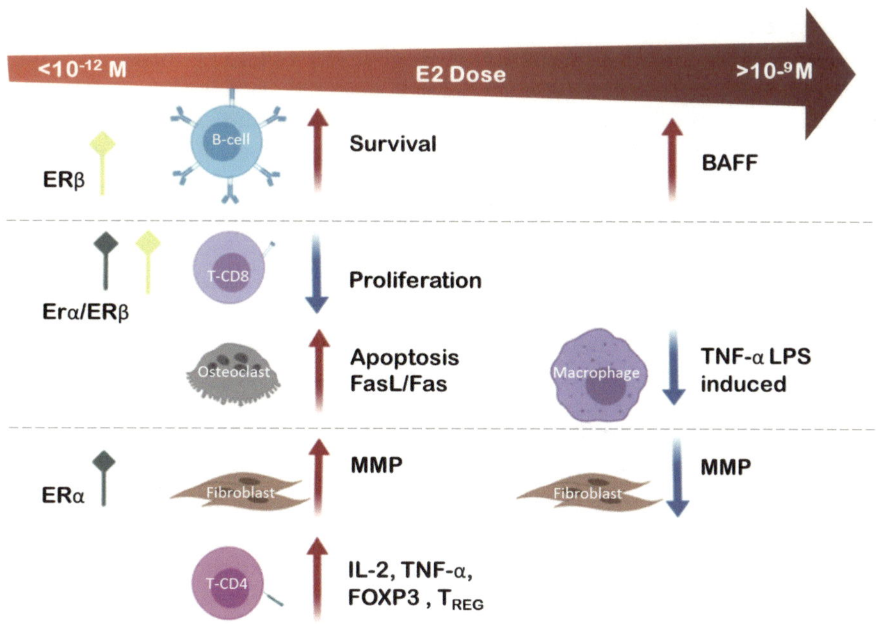

Figure 1.
E2 cell receptors in different cell populations: different effects of estrogen concentrations upon estrogen receptors ER-α and ER-β present on each cell. Left: receptors and cells were they are present. Horizontal red arrow: gradient of estrogen concentrations. Blue arrows: decrease of an effect by estrogen concentration. Red arrows: increase of an effect by estrogen concentrations. This is an original image made explicitly for this publication and not subject to copyright.

Another field with scarce exploration and understudied outcome of the estrogen therapy on RA is the modification and decrease of autoantibodies by estrogen action. This novel mechanism is not clearly elucidated and a lot of investigation in this topic is needed, but the little existing evidence demonstrate that estrogens can influence antibodies production and activity by modification of glycosylation of antibodies like galactosylation of human IgG in healthy individuals [89]. The changes in immunogenesis of antibodies by estrogens was demonstrated in an experiment were the induction of anti-C11 autoantibodies was measured, lower anti-C11 levels were observed in the estrogen treated group as compared with their controls [90]. The same behavior was observed by Nielsen et al. [91] and further investigations demonstrated than on CIA models sustained levels of 0.36 mg of estradiol (comparable to estrus phase) had similar quantities of IgG anti-CII antibodies than controls but have not developed RA, this was due to the different Ig subclasses. Estradiol-treated mice produced more IgG1, and mice from the placebo group produced significantly higher levels of IgG3 [92]. Other changes that estrogens induce in autoantibodies are an increase in sialylation, which has been observed during pregnancy and within 3 months post-delivery (when RA risk is presumably higher) [93]. Antibodies sialylation affects inflammation; in the case of RA, the transition from preclinical asymptomatic autoimmunity to clinical phases is associated with a change in the sialylation of antibodies [94–96]. Changes in sialylation by estrogens have been explored already in RA patients. E2 treatment increases sialylation on postmenopausal RA women [97], so taken together if E2 induces anti-inflammatory IgG by inducing St6Gal1 expression in antibody-producing cells [98].

4.3 Estrogen effects: dependency on concentration and chemical modifications

Estrogen concentration: it seems to exist a cut-off point in the concentration of estrogens that determine different effects, because sensitivity of receptors even at sub physiological concentrations of estrogens. For example, in a model of collagen-induced arthritis (CIA) in female mice, after type II collagen (CII) immunization those treated with the ER antagonist ICI 182,780 (which binds to both ERα and ERβ but not to the surface receptor) doses that insufficient to block estrus cycle, were sufficient for block the E3-mediated suppression of CIA [99, 100]. On the range of higher concentrations, estradiol (E2) can inhibit the production of pro-inflammatory cytokines, like TNF-α, (IL)-1 β, and IL-6 and induce anti-inflammatory cytokines such as IL-4, IL-10, and TGF-β (Th2 phenotype). On the contrary, low concentration of E2 stimulates TNF, INF-γ, and IL-1 β production and exerts an inhibitor effect on NK cells [101, 102]. In brain tissue, it was demonstrated that 2-OH-estradiol protects neurons from oxidative stress at nanomolar concentrations (10 nmol/L) but 17-β-estradiol showed oxidative effects only at micromolar concentrations (1–10 μmol/L); these concentrations were in the order of magnitude expected to activate their receptors (10–1000 nmol/L) demonstrating that physiological levels of estradiol may protect through receptor-dependent mechanisms from mitochondrial ROS, whereas higher concentrations may act through independent ER mechanisms [103]. This wide range of dose dependent effects could suggest us that a difference exists in the actions of estrogens between reproductive organs and its effects in the immune system. With respect to pro inflammatory cytokines such as TNF-αβ IL-1 and IL-6, estrogen effects seem to be bimodal where pharmacological concentrations (**Table 3**) of 50,000–100,000 pg/ml (equivalent to 100 μg/L or 10^{-6} M) decrease or inhibit the cytokine production and physiological concentrations of 5000 pg/ml increase cytokine production [104, 105]; this agree with other results where macrophages treated with doses of 0.001–100 nM

(10^{-9} M) equivalent to therapeutic concentrations of estradiol for 24 reduced LPS-induced TNF-α production [106]. Despite all evidence there is no clear explanation about how estrogens (estradiol or estriol) interfere in the clinical outcomes and immune response in RA depending on ERα/ERβ or evidence of the effects associated to a certain dose range. This could be useful for the development of more selective ERα or ERβ agonists and antagonists.

Estrogen chemical modifications: as mentioned before, a correlation exists between estrogen concentration in synovial fluid and serum estrogens ($R = 0.79$, $P < 0.0003$), and concentration of free estrogens (E2) is higher in RA as compared to controls [13–15]. Therefore, measured estrogen concentration in synovia could reflect a general overview of estrogen body concentrations. There is a significantly higher level of androstenedione (a precursor of estrone and estradiol) in synovial fluid of RA patients as estrone (E1), suggesting that these higher levels are the result of an elevated activity of aromatase [14]. Available steroid pre-hormones are rapidly converted to estrogens, which seems to have pro-inflammatory activity in the synovial tissue. When analyzed more in detail, it was found that increased estrogen concentrations in RA synovial fluid (in women as in men) were 16α-hydroxyestrone and 4-hydroxyestradiol (hydroxylated forms), while the estrone levels were detected increased on RA patients, the 2-hydroxyestrone showed no differences comparing RA vs. healthy controls [14], and depending on its modifications, estrogens can trigger very different effect in the body. For example, the hydroxylated forms of estradiol, 16OH-E2 and 2OH-E2 enhance the proliferation of THP-1 (**Figure 2**) monocytes at high concentrations (10^{-9} M). Meanwhile, the hydroxylated estrones 4OH-E1 and 2OH-E1 enhance cell proliferation at low concentration (10^{-10} M), [107], which are inhibited by antiestrogen drugs [108], except for 2OH-E1, which still induced proliferative effect (10^{-10} M) [107]. In some cases, estrogens produce the same affect but have different target cells in a dose dependent manner because of the proportion of expression of ERs; E2 and endocrine disrupting chemicals (EDCs) affect cell mutagenesis through ERα. At 10–8 M is observed an inhibition on the mitogenesis of B cells and at 10–6 M in T cells. For the EDCs

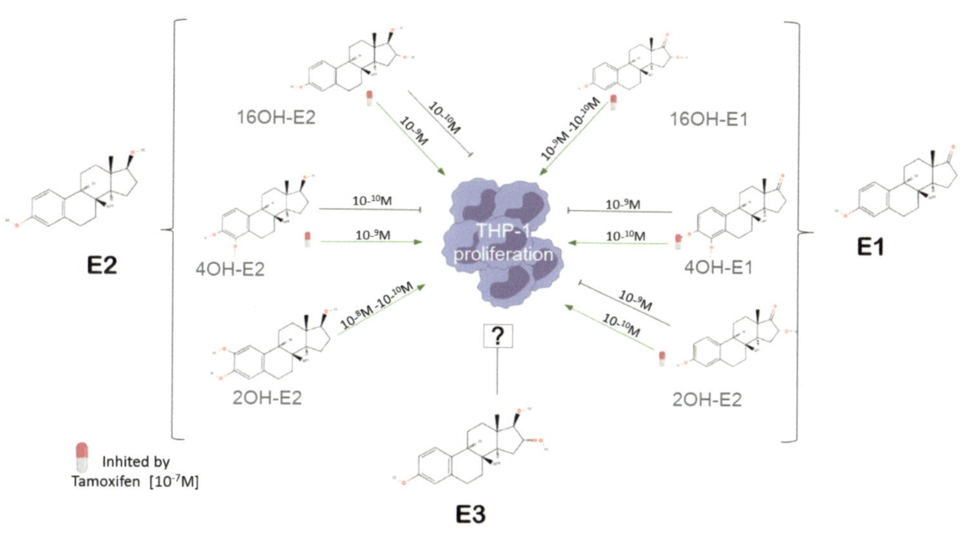

Figure 2.
Estrogen modifications and concentrations: image showing the differences between the effects depending of the estrogen modifications. Activity of different estrogen modifications upon proliferation of THP-1 cells and concentrations needed for achieve the effect. Green lines: increase in proliferation. Red lines: decrease in proliferation. This is an original image made explicitly for this publication and not subject to copyright.

(diethylstilbestrol, bisphenol-A, p-nonylphenol, and di-2-ethylhexylphthalate), the concentrations needed for this effect were higher, from 10 to 6 to 10–5 M [69].

5. Estrogens and their possible ameliorative effect upon arthritis: therapeutic approach

Given the previously displayed effects of estrogens on the immune system and in RA, it is natural to suppose that a hormone therapy could have certain effects upon the disease but, the studies exploring this possibility are scarce. Three major considerations have been identified as roadblock for such research to be conducted: (1) cut-off point in estrogen levels determining the effects of this molecule on the immune system, (2) the various effects of the same molecule at different concentrations lead to different effects depending ERα or ERβ receptor, and (3) effects dependent of the chemical modification (hydroxylation) of estrogens.

The hypothesis that hormonal therapy could ameliorate RA arises from the evidence of reported improvement in multiple pregnancies and contraceptive use [109], but this evidence became more solid when the estrogen at physiological levels administration in models of type II collagen-induced arthritis model (CIA) ameliorated arthritis and suppressed T-cell-dependent autoimmune reactions [52, 90]. In this experiment, female mice were implanted with E2 release devices, which induced a chronic estrous phase, the high doses of E2 caused a 35-day delay of the onset of RA disease but without affecting frequency and severity; this delay was reduced to 10 days with lower E2 concentrations of 25 days with physiological E3 proved to be as efficient as the high dose E2 causing a 25 day delay [90]. E3 seems to have more pronounced effects than E2; this estrogen E3 is mainly produced in pregnancy [51, 52]. In EAE models, it seems that the estrogen-mediated protection is dependent upon ERα. For example in EAE homozygous ERαKO treated with estriol, no protective effect was registered, while WT mice presented a significant decrease in disease severity and significant reductions in pro inflammatory cytokines TNF, IFNγ, IL-2, and an increase in levels of the Th2 cytokine IL-5 [110]. The effect of estrogens at interact with ERα receptor is not only limited to the immune response; in murine ovariectomized mice with estrogen treatment by pellet implantation, a dramatic increase in bone mass was observed. This was mediated by ERα-mediated apoptosis of osteoclasts through activating FasL/Fas signaling [111]. This could be an indicator that similar protective effects of estrogens may be present in immune cells due to the expression of ERα in CD4 + T lymphocytes.

Estrogens have been demonstrated to have anti-inflammatory activity. In CIA models, estrogen supplementation reduced paw inflammation efficiently and decreased paw volume by 48% ($P < 0{\cdot}01$) [91], but we need to be aware that the activity of several estrogens (E1, E2, E3, and E4) is different and it depends not only on the hormone itself but also by the specific disease or even the specific clinical profile of the patient that is taking them. 2-methoxyestradiol on CIA model (20 days after the injection of type II collagen) produce a significant decrease in the arthritis index compared with that in the control mice ($P < 0.05$) despite it was not as efficient as estradiol [112]. Despite this is the most tested estrogen among studies for its effect in RA, Estradiol E2, in clinical applications, shows several side effects such as: hypertension, increased coagulation, and cancer incidence but a feature that both share is that they are protective in experimental autoimmune encephalomyelitis (EAE) and CIA [113].

The clinical data available is scarce and most of the available trials only evaluate the protective effect of OCP (oral contraceptive pill) and hormone replacement therapy (HRP) for RA. In a study of association between postmenopausal hormone therapy (PMH) use and the risk of rheumatoid arthritis (RA) in a subset of the Epidemiological Investigation of RA (EIRA) study, the users of PMH had a decreased risk of ACPA-positive RA compared with never users, mainly with a combined therapy (estrogen plus progestagens), they propose that PMH use might reduce the risk of ACPA-positive RA in post-menopausal women over 50 years of age, but not of ACPA-negative RA [114].

Regarding the role of OCP use in RA, there is a theory which explains that recent decrease in incidence of RA in women in the past 50 years may be in part due to increased use of the OCP, even when may be confounded by OC use being related to pregnancy avoidance and high social class [115]. During a 14 month period, 23,000 women who were using oral contraceptives were recruited, and a similar number of those who had never used OCP as controls and evaluated every 6 month intervals. Patients were classified as "current user," "former user," and "never user." The cases were categorized according to the woman's contraceptive status at the time of RA diagnosis (event). The trend for former users was $\chi 2 = 5.7$, ($p < 0.02$) and for the never users $\chi 2 = 15.0$, ($p < 0.01$) but the current users $\chi 2 = 0–85$, ($p > 005$) and for those who were aged 40–44 years at diagnosis had a significantly lower risk of rheumatoid arthritis than similarly aged never users (relative risk 0.29). At the end of the follow-up, women who were using the pill at the time of diagnosis had a statistically non-significant 20% reduction in their risk of rheumatoid arthritis but early in the study current users had a significant 50% risk reduction [116]. The same cohort was classified in groups of "takers" and "never takers" and was analyzed too for the incidence of RA. The standardized rate for takers was 49% of the control rate ($p < 0.01$) and resulted interesting an observed tendency for an increased incidence of RA forward 35 years; this tendency was conserved only in the group of "never takers" and suppressed in the takers [117].

wIn the Swedish EIRA study (population-based case-control) including 2641 cases and 4251 controls participants were questioned about OCP (oral contraceptive pill) full term need to be mentioned consumption, and potential confounders in order to calculate the ORs adjusted for age, residential area, smoking, and alcohol consumption. Compared with never users, the OCP users had a decreased risk of ACPA-positive RA (OR = 0.84) (95% CI 0.74–0.96) compared to the never users. Also the consumption for more than 7 years decreased the risk of both ACPA-positive ($p = 0.0037$) and ACPA-negative RA ($p = 0.0356$) compared to never users of OCP [118].

Most of the studies agree that the current or ever use of the OCP has a protective effect against RA, probably more delaying the onset rather than a preventing RA. But until now there is not a final conclusion because even the meta-analysis results are contradictory. In the meta-analysis of six case-control and three longitudinal studies, the overall pooled odds ratio of the studies was 0.73 for the adjusted results (95% CI 0.61–0.85) with the conclusion that OCP consumption prevents the progression to severe disease by modifying the disease process [119]. On the contrary in a meta-analysis performed by Qi et al. in 2014, the authors identified 1116 publications in PubMed and EMBASE databases. The meta-analysis of 12 case-control and 5 cohort studies were analyzed. Potential publication bias was evaluated using Begg's funnel plots and quantified by the Egger's test, as a sensitivity analysis was performed to investigate the influence of potential confounding factors like age, smoking, parity/pregnancy, body mass index, and social class on risk of develop RA. Here, no statistically significant association was observed between oral contraceptives and RA risk (RR = 0.88, 95% CI = 0.75–1.03) concluding that OCP consumption was not significantly associated with RA risk [120].

HRT (hormone replacement therapy) has been studied in regard to RA new-onset. On a study in a prospective cohort of 31,336 Iowa women (from 55 to

69 years) followed up during 11 years, 158 incident cases of RA were registered. Of the factors that showed an inverse association with RA, the authors identified pregnancy (P trend =0.01) and age at menopause (P trend =0.03), whereas polycystic ovary syndrome (relative risk [RR], 2.58; 95% confidence interval [CI], 1.06–6.30), endometriosis (RR, 1.72; 95% CI, 0.93–3.18), and hormone replacement therapy (RR, 1.47; 95% CI, 1.04–2.06) were positively associated with RA. If HRT is administered before RA is associated with a higher risk of developing the disease, studies suggest that when HRT is administered during RA, they have a favorable effect. In 88 postmenopausal women with RA who received HRT, vitamin D3, and calcium supplementation or vitamin D3 and calcium supplementation alone for 2 years, HRT use had a significant effect upon active RA, ameliorating effects on inflammation (ESR $p = 0.025$) DAS28 ($p = 0.036$) and was associated with slower progression of radiological joint destruction ($p = 0.026$) [121]. The continuous hormonal therapy given to suppress menstruation for regulation of menstrual bleeding, pelvic pain, and dysmenorrhea seems to have demonstrated improvement in RA [122].

6. Novel hormone analogs in RA

Recently, novel hormone analogs have been developed. ERB-041 is a selective ERβ agonist and has showed interesting effects in several inflammatory rodent models, including endometriosis, rheumatoid arthritis, inflammatory bowel, and sepsis [123, 124] where a strong effect on reduction of inflammation was observed. This selective effect was the antecedent for the development of other ERβ agonists like MF101 [125] that could be useful to modulate the inflammation and cytokine production in RA. No clinical trial data on these molecules have been published so far.

7. Conclusions

Given the higher prevalence of RA cases that occur in women, is natural to suspect that such differences are due to sexual hormones, specifically estrogens, which have been explored as part of pathophysiology, development, and progression of RA disease. Antecedents point to estrogens as strong modulators of immune response and function associated to RA. The role that sex hormones play in the development, cell activation, and alterations in immune function in autoimmune diseases is still a matter of intense research. The administration of estrogens may have a protective effect on RA development or in the onset of disease, delaying it. Also, experimental evidence suggests that estrogens demonstrated anti-inflammatory activity in animal models of RA. Such effects are mediated by modifications in antibody production and in post-translational modification of antibodies like sialylation (addition of syalic acid), involved on increased risk of RA in conditions with low estrogen levels such as menopause. Estrogens administration to RA patients could be a strategy to improve the quality of life through hormone replacement therapy (HRT). This, in resource limited settings were biological therapy cannot be afforded and in patients that are refractory to standard MTX therapy or that have failed to respond to such therapies.

Acknowledgements

Maria Fernanda Romo García thanks CONACyT (Consejo Nacional de Ciencia y Tecnologia); National Council of Science and Technology for scholarship 297364/ CVU 560269.

Conflict of interest

No conflict of interest is declared.

Author details

Maria Fernanda Romo-García[1,2], Martín Zapata-Zuñiga[3,4,5],
José Antonio Enciso-Moreno[1] and Julio Enrique Castañeda-Delgado[1,6*]

1 Cátedras-CONACyT-Unidad de Investigación Biomédica de Zacatecas, IMSS, Zacatecas, México

2 Departamento de Inmunología, Facultad de Medicina, Universidad Autónoma de San Luis Potosí, San Luis Potosí, México

3 Hospital Rural # 51, IMSS, Villanueva, Zacatecas, México

4 Hospital General Jerez Zacatecas, Servicios de Salud de Zacatecas, Zacatecas, México

5 Facultad de Medicina Humana y Ciencias de la Salud, Universidad Autónoma de Zacatecas, Zacatecas, México

6 Cátedras-CONACyT-Unidad de Investigación Biomédica de Zacatecas-IMSS, Zacatecas, México

*Address all correspondence to: julioenrique_castaeda@yahoo.com.mx

References

[1] Pelaez-Ballestas I, Sanin LH, Moreno-Montoya J, Alvarez-Nemegyei J, Burgos-Vargas R, Garza-Elizondo M, et al. Epidemiology of the rheumatic diseases in Mexico. A study of 5 regions based on the COPCORD methodology. The Journal of Rheumatology. 2011;**86**: 3-8. Available from: http://www.jrheum.org/cgi/doi/10.3899/jrheum.100951 [cited 14 December 2016]

[2] Alamanos Y, Voulgari PV, Drosos AA. Incidence and prevalence of rheumatoid arthritis, based on the 1987 American College of Rheumatology Criteria: A systematic review. Seminars in Arthritis and Rheumatism. 2006; **36**(3):182-188. Available from: http://www.ncbi.nlm.nih.gov/pubmed/17045630 [cited 18 September 2018]

[3] Szekanecz Z, Soós L, Szabó Z, Fekete A, Kapitány A, Végvári A, et al. Anti-citrullinated protein antibodies in rheumatoid arthritis: As good as it gets? Clinical Reviews in Allergy & Immunology. 2008;**34**(1):26-31. Available from: http://www.ncbi.nlm.nih.gov/pubmed/18270854 [cited 14 September 2017]

[4] Weyand CM, Klimiuk PA, Goronzy JJ. Heterogeneity of rheumatoid arthritis: From phenotypes to genotypes. Seminars in Immunopathology. 1998;**20** (1–2):5-22. Available from: http://link.springer.com/10.1007/BF00831996 [cited 30 October 2018]

[5] van der Pouw KTCTM, Wijbrandts CA, van Baarsen LGM, Voskuyl AE, Rustenburg F, Baggen JM, et al. Rheumatoid arthritis subtypes identified by genomic profiling of peripheral blood cells: Assignment of a type I interferon signature in a subpopulation of patients. Annals of the Rheumatic Diseases. 2007;**66**(8): 1008-1014. Available from: http://www.ncbi.nlm.nih.gov/pubmed/17223656 [cited 12 January 2018]

[6] Courvoisier DS, Alpizar-Rodriguez D, Gottenberg JE, Hernandez MV, Iannone F, Lie E, et al. Rheumatoid arthritis patients after initiation of a new biologic agent: Trajectories of disease activity in a large multinational cohort study. EBioMedicine. 2016;**11**:302-306. Available from: http://www.ncbi.nlm.nih.gov/pubmed/27558858 [cited 30 October 2018]

[7] Leitman DC, Paruthiyil S, Vivar OI, Saunier EF, Herber CB, Cohen I, et al. Regulation of specific target genes and biological responses by estrogen receptor subtype agonists. Current Opinion in Pharmacology. 2010;**10**(6): 629-636. Available from: http://www.ncbi.nlm.nih.gov/pubmed/20951642 [cited 14 August 2018]

[8] Ps H. The ameliorating effect of pregnancy on chronic atrophic (infectious rheumatoid) arthritis, fibrositis, and intermittent hydrarthrosis. Proceedings of the Staff Meetings. Mayo Clinic. 1938;**13**:161-167

[9] Nolten WE, Lindheimer MD, RUECKERT PA, Oparil S, Ehrlich EN. Diurnal patterns and regulation of cortisol secretion in pregnancy. The Journal of Clinical Endocrinology & Metabolism. 1980;**51**(3):466-472. Available from: http://www.ncbi.nlm.nih.gov/pubmed/7410530 [cited 12 September 2018]

[10] Deighton CM, Watson MJ, Walker DJ. Sex hormones in postmenopausal HLA-identical rheumatoid arthritis discordant sibling pairs. The Journal of Rheumatology. 1992;**19**(11):1663-1667. Available from: http://www.ncbi.nlm.nih.gov/pubmed/1491383 [cited 28 September 2018]

[11] Hall GM, Perry LA, Spector TD. Depressed levels of dehydroepiandrosterone sulphate in postmenopausal women with rheumatoid arthritis but no

relation with axial bone density. Annals of the Rheumatic Diseases. 1993;**52**(3): 211-214. Available from: http://www.ncbi.nlm.nih.gov/pubmed/8484674 [cited 28 September 2018]

[12] Cash JM, Crofford LJ, Gallucci WT, Sternberg EM, Gold PW, Chrousos GP, et al. Pituitary-adrenal axis responsiveness to ovine corticotropin releasing hormone in patients with rheumatoid arthritis treated with low dose prednisone. The Journal of Rheumatology. 1992;**19**(11):1692-1696. Available from: http://www.ncbi.nlm.nih.gov/pubmed/1337108 [cited 28 September 2018]

[13] Cutolo M, Villaggio B, Craviotto C, Pizzorni C, Seriolo B, Sulli A. Sex hormones and rheumatoid arthritis. Autoimmunity Reviews. 2002;**1**(5): 284-289. Available from: https://www.sciencedirect.com/science/article/pii/S1568997202000642?via%3Dihub [cited 18 September 2018]

[14] Castagnetta LA, Carruba G, Granata OM, Stefano R, Miele M, Schmidt M, et al. Increased estrogen formation and estrogen to androgen ratio in the synovial fluid of patients with rheumatoid arthritis. The Journal of Rheumatology. 2003;**30**(12): 2597-2605. Available from: http://www.ncbi.nlm.nih.gov/pubmed/14719200 [cited 18 September 2018]

[15] Richette P, Laborde K, Boutron C, Bardin T, Corvol M-T, Savouret J-F. Correlation between serum and synovial fluid estrogen concentrations: Comment on the article by Sowers et al. Arthritis & Rheumatology. 2007;**56**(2):698-698. Available from: http://doi.wiley.com/10.1002/art.22384

[16] Abbassi-Ghanavati M, Greer LG, Cunningham FG. Pregnancy and laboratory studies. Obstetrics & Gynecology. 2009;**114**(6):1326-1331. Available from: http://www.ncbi.nlm.nih.gov/pubmed/19935037 [cited 03 October 2018]

[17] Altemus M, Deuster PA, Galliven E, Carter CS, Gold PW. Suppression of hypothalmic-pituitary-adrenal axis responses to stress in lactating women. The Journal of Clinical Endocrinology and Metabolism. 1995;**80**(10):2954-2959

[18] Jacobson DL, Gange SJ, Rose NR, Graham NM. Epidemiology and estimated population burden of selected autoimmune diseases in the United States. Clinical Immunology and Immunopathology. 1997;**84**(3):223-243. Available from: http://www.ncbi.nlm.nih.gov/pubmed/9281381 [cited 29 October 2018]

[19] Fairweather D, Rose NR. Women and autoimmune diseases. Emerging Infectious Diseases. 2004;**10**(11): 2005-2011. Available from: http://www.ncbi.nlm.nih.gov/pubmed/15550215 [cited 29 October 2018]

[20] Wolfe AM, Kellgren JH, Masi AT. The epidemiology of rheumatoid arthritis: A review. II. Incidence and diagnostic criteria. Bulletin on the Rheumatic Diseases. 1968;**19**(3): 524-529. Available from: http://www.ncbi.nlm.nih.gov/pubmed/4884388 [cited 29 October 2018]

[21] van Vollenhoven RF. Sex differences in rheumatoid arthritis: More than meets the eye. BMC Medicine. 2009;**7**(1):12. Available from: http://bmcmedicine.biomedcentral.com/articles/10.1186/1741-7015-7-12 [cited 21 September 2018]

[22] Forslind K, Hafström I, Ahlmén M, Svensson B, BARFOT Study Group. Sex: A major predictor of remission in early rheumatoid arthritis? Annals of the Rheumatic Diseases. 2007;**66**(1):46-52. Available from: http://www.ncbi.nlm.nih.gov/pubmed/17158139 [cited 19 September 2018]

[23] Couderc M, Gottenberg J-E, Mariette X, Pereira B, Bardin T, Cantagrel A, et al. Influence of gender on response to rituximab in patients with rheumatoid arthritis: Results from the autoimmunity and rituximab registry. Rheumatology. 2014;**53**(10): 1788-1793. Available from: https://academic.oup.com/rheumatology/article-lookup/doi/10.1093/rheumatology/keu176 [cited 21 September 2018]

[24] Sokka T, Toloza S, Cutolo M, Kautiainen H, Makinen H, Gogus F, et al. Women, men, and rheumatoid arthritis: Analyses of disease activity, disease characteristics, and treatments in the QUEST-RA study. Arthritis Research & Therapy. 2009;**11**(1):R7. Available from: http://www.ncbi.nlm.nih.gov/pubmed/19144159 [cited 03 September 2018]

[25] Alpízar-Rodríguez D, Pluchino N, Canny G, Gabay C, Finckh A. The role of female hormonal factors in the development of rheumatoid arthritis. Rheumatology. 2016;**56**(8):kew318. Available from: https://academic.oup.com/rheumatology/article-lookup/doi/10.1093/rheumatology/kew318 [cited 31 October 2018]

[26] Chen H, Zhu H, Zhang K, Chen K, Yang H. Estrogen deficiency accelerates lumbar facet joints arthritis. Scientific Reports. 2017;**7**(1):1379. Available from: http://www.nature.com/articles/s41598-017-01427-7 [cited 31 October 2018]

[27] Merlino LA, Cerhan JR, Criswell LA, Mikuls TR, Saag KG. Estrogen and other female reproductive risk factors are not strongly associated with the development of rheumatoid arthritis in elderly women. Semin Arthritis Rheum. September 2003;**33**(2):72-82

[28] Sinaii N, Cleary SD, Ballweg ML, Nieman LK, Stratton P. High rates of autoimmune and endocrine disorders, fibromyalgia, chronic fatigue syndrome and atopic diseases among women with endometriosis: A survey analysis. Human Reproduction. 2002;**17**(10): 2715-2724. Available from: http://www.ncbi.nlm.nih.gov/pubmed/12351553 [cited 24 September 2018]

[29] Lleo A, Battezzati PM, Selmi C, Gershwin ME, Podda M. Is autoimmunity a matter of sex? Autoimmunity Reviews. 2008;**7**(8): 626-630. Available from: http://www.ncbi.nlm.nih.gov/pubmed/18603021 [cited 03 September 2018]

[30] Häupl T, Østensen M, Grützkau A, Radbruch A, Burmester G-R, Villiger PM. Reactivation of rheumatoid arthritis after pregnancy increased phagocyte and recurring lymphocyte gene activity. Arthritis & Rheumatology. 2008;**58**(10):2981-2992. Avaielable from: https://onlinelibrary.wiley.com/doi/pdf/10.1002/art.23907 [cited 06 September 2018]

[31] Kanik KS, Wilder RL. Hormonal alterations in rheumatoid arthritis, including the effects of pregnancy. Rheumatic Disease Clinics of North America. 2000;**26**(4):805-823. Available from: http://linkinghub.elsevier.com/retrieve/pii/S0889857X05701708

[32] Barrett JH, Brennan P, Fiddler M, Silman AJ. Does rheumatoid arthritis remit during pregnancy and relapse postpartum?: Results from a nationwide study in the United Kingdom performed prospectively from late pregnancy. Arthritis & Rheumatology. 1999;**42**(6): 1219-1227. Available from: http://www.ncbi.nlm.nih.gov/pubmed/10366115 [cited 06 September 2018]

[33] Iijima T, Tada H, Hidaka Y, Yagoro A, Mitsuda N, Kanzaki T, et al. Prediction of postpartum onset of rheumatoid arthritis. Annals of the Rheumatic Diseases. 1998;**57**:460-463. Available from: http://ard.bmj.com/ [cited 06 September 2018]

[34] Ostensen M, Fuhrer L, Mathieu R, Seitz M, Villiger PM. A prospective study of pregnant patients with

rheumatoid arthritis and ankylosing spondylitis using validated clinical instruments. Annals of the Rheumatic Diseases. 2004;**63**(10):1212-1217. Available from: http://www.ncbi.nlm.nih.gov/pubmed/15361373 [cited 12 September 2018]

[35] Oka M. Effect of pregnancy on the onset and course of rheumatoid arthritis. Obstetrical and Gynecological Survey. 1954;**9**(2):180-181. Available from: http://ard.bmj.com/ [cited 13 September 2018]

[36] Del Junco DJ, Annegers JF, Coulam CB, Luthra HS. The relationship between rheumatoid arthritis and reproductive function. British Journal of Rheumatology. 1989;**28** (Suppl 1):33; discussion 42-5. Available from: http://www.ncbi.nlm.nih.gov/pubmed/2819346 [cited 13 September 2018]

[37] Nelson JL, Ostensen M. Pregnancy and rheumatoid arthritis. Rheumatic Disease Clinics of North America. 1997; **23**(1):195-212. Available from: http://www.ncbi.nlm.nih.gov/pubmed/9031383 [cited 06 September 2018]

[38] Silman A, Kay A, Brennan P. Timing of pregnancy in relation to the onset of rheumatoid arthritis. Arthritis & Rheumatology. 1992;**35**(2):152-155. Available from: http://www.ncbi.nlm.nih.gov/pubmed/1734904 [cited 12 September 2018]

[39] Skomsvoll JF, Ostensen M, Irgens LM, Baste V. Pregnancy complications and delivery practice in women with connective tissue disease and inflammatory rheumatic disease in Norway. Acta Obstetricia et Gynecologica Scandinavica. 2000;**79**(6): 490-495. Available from: http://www.ncbi.nlm.nih.gov/pubmed/10857874 [cited 12 September 2018]

[40] Jara LJ, Medina G, Saavedra MA, Vera-Lastra O, Navarro C. Prolactin and autoimmunity. Clinical Reviews in Allergy and Immunology. 2011;**40**(1): 50-59

[41] Shelly S, Boaz M, Orbach H. Prolactin and autoimmunity. Autoimmunity Reviews. 2012;**11**(6–7): A465-A470. Available from: http://www.ncbi.nlm.nih.gov/pubmed/22155203 [cited 12 September 2018]

[42] Brennan P, Silman A. Breast-feeding and the onset of rheumatoid arthritis. Arthritis & Rheumatology. 1994;**37**(6):808-813. Available from: http://www.ncbi.nlm.nih.gov/pubmed/8003052 [cited 12 September 2018]

[43] Mor G, Cardenas I, Abrahams V, Guller S. Inflammation and pregnancy: The role of the immune system at the implantation site. Annals of the New York Academy of Sciences. 2011; **1221**(1):80-87. Available from: http://www.ncbi.nlm.nih.gov/pubmed/21401634 [cited 13 September 2018]

[44] Steiner M, Haskett RF, Carroll BJ. Premenstrual tension syndrome: The development of research diagnostic criteria and new rating scales. Acta Psychiatrica Scandinavica. 1980;**62**(2): 177-190. Available from: http://www.ncbi.nlm.nih.gov/pubmed/7193399 [cited 20 September 2018]

[45] Rudge SR, Kowanko IC, Drury PL, Bartholomew S. Menstrual cyclicity of finger joint size and grip strength in patients with rheumatoid arthritis. Annals of the Rheumatic Diseases. August 1983; **42**(4):425-430. Available from: http://ard.bmj.com/ [cited 20 September 2018]

[46] Latman NS. Relation of menstrual cycle phase to symptoms of rheumatoid arthritis. The American Journal of Medicine. 1983;**74**(6):957-960. Available from: http://linkinghub.elsevier.com/retrieve/pii/0002934383907891 [cited 21 September 2018]

[47] McDonagh JE, Singh MM, Griffiths ID, McDonagh ID, Griffiths JE. Menstrual arthritis. Annals of the

Rheumatic Diseases. 1993;**52**:65-66. Available from: http://ard.bmj.com/ [cited 20 September 2018]

[48] Østensen M, Villiger PM. The remission of rheumatoid arthritis during pregnancy. Seminars in Immunopathology. 2007;**29**(2):185-191. Available from: http://www.ncbi.nlm.nih.gov/pubmed/17621703 [cited 03 September 2018]

[49] Krause ML, Makol A. Management of rheumatoid arthritis during pregnancy: Challenges and solutions. Open Access Rheumatology: Research and Reviews. 2016;**8**:23-36. Available from: http://www.ncbi.nlm.nih.gov/pubmed/27843367 [cited 03 September 2018]

[50] de Man YA, Dolhain RJEM, van de Geijn FE, Willemsen SP, Hazes JMW. Disease activity of rheumatoid arthritis during pregnancy: Results from a nationwide prospective study. Arthritis & Rheumatology. 2008;**59**(9): 1241-1248. Available from: http://www.ncbi.nlm.nih.gov/pubmed/18759316 [cited 06 September 2018]

[51] Jansson L, Holmdahl R. Estrogen-mediated immunosuppression in autoimmune diseases. Inflammation Research. 1998;**47**(7):290-301. Available from: http://www.ncbi.nlm.nih.gov/pubmed/9719493 [cited 18 September 2018]

[52] Jansson L, Olsson T, Holmdahl R. Estrogen induces a potent suppression of experimental autoimmune encephalomyelitis and collagen-induced arthritis in mice. Journal of Neuroimmunology. 1994;**53**(2):203-207. Available from: http://www.ncbi.nlm.nih.gov/pubmed/8071434 [cited 18 September 2018]

[53] Holinka CF, Diczfalusy E, Coelingh Bennink HJT. Estetrol: A unique steroid in human pregnancy. Journal of Steroid Biochemistry and Molecular Biology. 2008;**110**(1–2):138-143. Available from: http://www.ncbi.nlm.nih.gov/pubmed/18462934 [cited 08 October 2018]

[54] Groen B, van der Wijk A-E, van den Berg PP, Lefrandt JD, van den Berg G, Sollie KM, et al. Immunological adaptations to pregnancy in women with type 1 diabetes. Scientific Reports. 2015;**5**:13618. Available from: http://www.ncbi.nlm.nih.gov/pubmed/26391604 [cited 12 September 2018]

[55] Veenstra van Nieuwenhoven AL, Heineman MJ, Faas MM. The immunology of successful pregnancy. Human Reproduction Update. 2003; **9**(4):347-357. Available from: http://www.ncbi.nlm.nih.gov/pubmed/12926528 [cited 12 September 2018]

[56] Russell AS, Johnston C, Chew C, Maksymowych WP. Evidence for reduced Th1 function in normal pregnancy: A hypothesis for the remission of rheumatoid arthritis. The Journal of Rheumatology. 1997;**24**(6): 1045-1050. Available from: http://www.ncbi.nlm.nih.gov/pubmed/9195507

[57] Aluvihare VR, Kallikourdis M, Betz AG. Regulatory T cells mediate maternal tolerance to the fetus. Nature Immunology. 2004;**5**(3):266-271. Available from: http://www.ncbi.nlm.nih.gov/pubmed/14758358 [cited 13 September 2018]

[58] Bulmer JN, Pace D, Ritson A. Immunoregulatory cells in human decidua: Morphology, immunohistochemistry and function. Reproduction Nutrition Development. 1988;**28**(6B):1599-1613. Available from: http://www.ncbi.nlm.nih.gov/pubmed/3073448 [cited 13 September 2018]

[59] Shimada S, Nishida R, Takeda M, Iwabuchi K, Kishi R, Onoe K, et al. Natural killer, natural killer T, helper and cytotoxic T cells in the decidua from sporadic miscarriage. American Journal of Reproductive Immunology. 2006; **56**(3):193-200. Available from: http://

doi.wiley.com/10.1111/j.1600-0897.2006.00417.x [cited 13 September 2018]

[60] Colangelo K, Haig S, Bonner A, Zelenietz C, Pope J. Self-reported flaring varies during the menstrual cycle in systemic lupus erythematosus compared with rheumatoid arthritis and fibromyalgia. Rheumatology. 2011; **50**(4):703-708. Available from: https://academic.oup.com/rheumatology/article-lookup/doi/10.1093/rheumatology/keq360 [cited 19 September 2018]

[61] Costenbader KH, Feskanich D, Stampfer MJ, Karlson EW. Reproductive and menopausal factors and risk of systemic lupus erythematosus in women. Arthritis & Rheumatology. 2007;**56**(4):1251-1262. Available from: http://www.ncbi.nlm.nih.gov/pubmed/17393454 [cited 24 September 2018]

[62] Thomas C, Gustafsson JÅ. The different roles of ER subtypes in cancer biology and therapy. Nature Reviews Cancer. 22 July 2011;**11**(8):597-608. DOI: 10.1038/nrc3093

[63] Tee MK, Rogatsky I, Tzagarakis-Foster C, Cvoro A, An J, Christy RJ, et al. Estradiol and selective estrogen receptor modulators differentially regulate target genes with estrogen receptors alpha and beta. Molecular Biology of the Cell. 2004;**15**(3):1262-1272. Available from: http://www.ncbi.nlm.nih.gov/pubmed/14699072 [cited 03 September 2018]

[64] Stossi F, Barnett DH, Frasor J, Komm B, Lyttle CR, Katzenellenbogen BS. Transcriptional profiling of estrogen-regulated gene expression via estrogen receptor (ER) α or ERβ in human osteosarcoma cells: Distinct and common target genes for these receptors. Endocrinology. 2004; **145**(7):3473-3486. Available from: http://www.ncbi.nlm.nih.gov/pubmed/15033914 [cited 03 September 2018]

[65] Paruthiyil S, Cvoro A, Zhao X, Wu Z, Sui Y, Staub RE, et al. Drug and cell type-specific regulation of genes with different classes of estrogen receptor β-selective agonists. PLOS One. 2009;**4**(7):e6271. Laudet V, editor. Available from: http://www.ncbi.nlm.nih.gov/pubmed/19609440 [cited 03 September 2018]

[66] Phiel KL, Henderson RA, Adelman SJ, Elloso MM. Differential estrogen receptor gene expression in human peripheral blood mononuclear cell populations. Immunology Letters. 2005;**97**(1):107-113. Available from: https://www.sciencedirect.com/science/article/abs/pii/S0165247804002792 [cited 27 September 2018]

[67] Mao A, Paharkova-Vatchkova V, Hardy J, Miller MM, Kovats S. Estrogen selectively promotes the differentiation of dendritic cells with characteristics of Langerhans cells. The Journal of Immunology. 2005;**175**(8):5146-5151. Available from: http://www.ncbi.nlm.nih.gov/pubmed/16210618 [cited 20 September 2018]

[68] Curran EM, Berghaus LJ, Vernetti NJ, Saporita AJ, Lubahn DB, Estes DM. Natural killer cells express estrogen receptor-α and estrogen receptor-β and can respond to estrogen via a non-estrogen receptor-α-mediated pathway. Cellular Immunology. 2001; **214**(1):12-20. Available from: http://www.ncbi.nlm.nih.gov/pubmed/11902825 [cited 20 September 2018]

[69] Sakazaki H, Ueno H, Nakamuro K. Estrogen receptor alpha in mouse splenic lymphocytes: Possible involvement in immunity. Toxicology Letters. 2002;**133**(2–3):221-229. Available from: http://www.ncbi.nlm.nih.gov/pubmed/12119130 [cited 19 September 2018]

[70] Kovats S. Estrogen receptors regulate innate immune cells and

signaling pathways. Cellular Immunology. 2015;**294**(2):63-69. Available from: http://linkinghub.elsevier.com/retrieve/pii/S000887491500026X [cited 20 September 2018]

[71] Maret A, Coudert JD, Garidou L, Foucras G, Gourdy P, Krust A, et al. Estradiol enhances primary antigen-specific CD4 T cell responses and Th1 development in vivo. Essential role of estrogen receptor α expression in hematopoietic cells. European Journal of Immunology. 2003;**33**(2):512-521. Available from: http://doi.wiley.com/10.1002/immu.200310027 [cited 14 September 2018]

[72] Erlandsson MC, Ohlsson C, Gustafsson JA, Carlsten H. Role of oestrogen receptors alpha and beta in immune organ development and in oestrogen-mediated effects on thymus. Immunology. 2001;**103**(1):17-25. Available from: http://www.ncbi.nlm.nih.gov/pubmed/11380688 [cited 27 September 2018]

[73] Polanczyk MJ, Hopke C, Huan J, Vandenbark AA, Offner H. Enhanced FoxP3 expression and Treg cell function in pregnant and estrogen-treated mice. Journal of Neuroimmunology. 2005;**170**(1–2):85-92. Available from: http://www.ncbi.nlm.nih.gov/pubmed/16253347 [cited 18 September 2018]

[74] Tan IJ, Peeva E, Zandman-Goddard G. Hormonal modulation of the immune system — A spotlight on the role of progestogens. Autoimmunity Reviews. 2015;**14**(6):536-542. Available from: http://www.ncbi.nlm.nih.gov/pubmed/25697984 [cited 12 September 2018]

[75] Prieto GA, Rosenstein Y. Oestradiol potentiates the suppressive function of human CD4+ CD25+ regulatory T cells by promoting their proliferation. Immunology. 2006;**118**(1):58-65. Available from: http://www.ncbi.nlm.nih.gov/pubmed/16630023 [cited 19 September 2018]

[76] Arruvito L, Sanz M, Banham AH, Fainboim L. Expansion of CD4+CD25+and FOXP3+ regulatory T cells during the follicular phase of the menstrual cycle: Implications for human reproduction. The Journal of Immunology. 2007;**178**(4):2572-2578. Available from: http://www.ncbi.nlm.nih.gov/pubmed/17277167 [cited 19 September 2018]

[77] Lee S, Kim J, Jang B, Hur S, Jung U, Kil K, et al. Fluctuation of peripheral blood T, B, and NK cells during a menstrual cycle of normal healthy women. The Journal of Immunology. 2010;**185**(1):756-762. Available from: http://www.ncbi.nlm.nih.gov/pubmed/20530263 [cited 19 September 2018]

[78] Somerset DA, Zheng Y, Kilby MD, Sansom DM, Drayson MT. Normal human pregnancy is associated with an elevation in the immune suppressive CD25+ CD4+ regulatory T-cell subset. Immunology. 2004;**112**(1):38-43. Available from: http://www.ncbi.nlm.nih.gov/pubmed/15096182 [cited 19 September 2018]

[79] Josefsson E, Tarkowski A, Dahlin A-G, Crafoord F, Thuring I, Lundgren M, et al. Suppression of type I1 collagen-induced arthritis by the endogenous estrogen metabolite 2-methoxyestradiol [internet]. Arthritis and Rheumatism. 1997;**40**. Available from: https://onlinelibrary.wiley.com/doi/pdf/10.1002/art.1780400120 [cited 18 September 2018]

[80] Khalkhali-Ellis Z, Seftor EA, Nieva DR, Handa RJ, Price RH, Kirschmann DA, et al. Estrogen and progesterone regulation of human fibroblast-like synoviocyte function in vitro: Implications in rheumatoid arthritis. The Journal of Rheumatology. 2000;**27**(7):1622-1631. Available from: http://www.ncbi.nlm.nih.gov/pubmed/10914842 [cited 18 September 2018]

[81] Macdiarmid F, Wang D, Duncan LJ, Purohit A, Ghilchick MW, Reed MJ.

Stimulation of aromatase activity in breast fibroblasts by tumor necrosis factor alpha. Molecular and Cellular Endocrinology. 1994;**106**(1–2):17-21. Available from: http://www.ncbi.nlm.nih.gov/pubmed/7895904 [cited 18 September 2018]

[82] Grimaldi CM, Cleary J, Dagtas AS, Moussai D, Diamond B. Estrogen alters thresholds for B cell apoptosis and activation. The Journal of Clinical Investigation. 2002;**109**(12):1625-1633. Available from: http://www.ncbi.nlm.nih.gov/pubmed/12070310 [cited 19 September 2018]

[83] Grimaldi CM, Michael DJ, Diamond B. Cutting edge: Expansion and activation of a population of autoreactive marginal zone B cells in a model of estrogen-induced lupus. The Journal of Immunology. 2001;**167**(4):1886-1890. Available from: http://www.ncbi.nlm.nih.gov/pubmed/11489967 [cited 19 September 2018]

[84] Manuela D, Dalila S, Yara M, Souza Iliada LS. BAFF expression is modulated by female hormones in human immune cells. Biochemical Genetics. 2016;**54**(5):722-730. Available from: https://web.a.ebscohost.com/abstract?direct=true&profile=ehost&scope=site&authtype=crawler&jrnl=00062928&AN=118005841&h=oqMhwcHnmf8F6Nm4QzoiydPzgd2uvK%2FM1L02Uq3iC1h5Yib2LNu3PyDFDz8ZTfz5F16wIe3IhL3PgeVvFkJSig%3D%3D&crl=f&resultNs=AdminWebAuth&resultLocal= [cited 20 September 2018]

[85] Morimoto S, Nakano S, Watanabe T, Tamayama Y, Mitsuo A, Nakiri Y, et al. Expression of B-cell activating factor of the tumour necrosis factor family (BAFF) in T cells in active systemic lupus erythematosus: The role of BAFF in T cell-dependent B cell pathogenic autoantibody production. Rheumatology. 2007;**46**(7):1083-1086. Available from: http://www.ncbi.nlm.nih.gov/pubmed/17500077 [cited 20 September 2018]

[86] Eilertsen GØ, Van Ghelue M, Strand H, Nossent JC. Increased levels of BAFF in patients with systemic lupus erythematosus are associated with acute-phase reactants, independent of BAFF genetics: A case–control study. Rheumatology. 2011;**50**(12):2197-2205. Available from: https://academic.oup.com/rheumatology/article-lookup/doi/10.1093/rheumatology/ker282 [cited 20 September 2018]

[87] Bosello S, Youinou P, Daridon C, Tolusso B, Bendaoud B, Pietrapertosa D, et al. Concentrations of BAFF correlate with autoantibody levels, clinical disease activity, and response to treatment in early rheumatoid arthritis. The Journal of Rheumatology. 2008;**35**(7):1256-1264. Available from: http://www.ncbi.nlm.nih.gov/pubmed/18528969 [cited 20 September 2018]

[88] Peeva E, Venkatesh J, Diamond B. Tamoxifen blocks estrogen-induced B cell maturation but not survival. The Journal of Immunology. 2005;**175**(3):1415-1423. Available from: http://www.ncbi.nlm.nih.gov/pubmed/16034077 [cited 19 September 2018]

[89] Ercan A, Kohrt WM, Cui J, Deane KD, Pezer M, Yu EW, et al. Estrogens regulate glycosylation of IgG in women and men. JCI Insight. 2017;**2**(4):e89703. Available from: http://www.ncbi.nlm.nih.gov/pubmed/28239652 [cited 17 September 2018]

[90] Jansson L, Mattsson A, Mattsson R, Holmdahl R. Estrogen induced suppression of collagen arthritis V: Physiological level of estrogen in DBA1 mice is therapeutic on established arthritis, suppresses anti-type II collagen T-cell dependent immunity and stimulates polyclonal B-cell activity. Journal of Autoimmunity. 1990;**3**(3):257-270. Available from: https://www.sciencedirect.com/science/article/pii/089684119090145I [cited 18 September 2018]

[91] Nielsen RH, Christiansen C, Stolina M, Karsdal MA. Oestrogen exhibits type II collagen protective effects and attenuates collagen-induced arthritis in rats. Clinical & Experimental Immunology. 2008; **152**(1):21-27. Available from: http://www.ncbi.nlm.nih.gov/pubmed/18241229 [cited 18 September 2018]

[92] Latham KA, Zamora A, Drought H, Subramanian S, Matejuk A, Offner H, et al. Estradiol treatment redirects the isotype of the autoantibody response and prevents the development of autoimmune arthritis. The Journal of Immunology. 2003;**171**(11):5820-5827. Available from: http://www.ncbi.nlm.nih.gov/pubmed/14634091 [cited 14 September 2018]

[93] van de Geijn FE, Wuhrer M, Selman MH, Willemsen SP, de Man YA, Deelder AM, et al. Immunoglobulin G galactosylation and sialylation are associated with pregnancy-induced improvement of rheumatoid arthritis and the postpartum flare: Results from a large prospective cohort study. Arthritis Research & Therapy. 2009;**11**(6):R193. Available from: http://www.ncbi.nlm.nih.gov/pubmed/20015375 [cited 17 September 2018]

[94] Böhm S, Schwab I, Lux A, Nimmerjahn F. The role of sialic acid as a modulator of the anti-inflammatory activity of IgG. Seminars in Immunopathology. 2012;**34**(3):443-453. Available from: http://www.ncbi.nlm.nih.gov/pubmed/22437760 [cited 17 September 2018]

[95] Rombouts Y, Ewing E, van de Stadt LA, Selman MHJ, Trouw LA, Deelder AM, et al. Anti-citrullinated protein antibodies acquire a pro-inflammatory Fc glycosylation phenotype prior to the onset of rheumatoid arthritis. Annals of the Rheumatic Diseases. 2015;**74**(1): 234-241. Available from: http://www.ncbi.nlm.nih.gov/pubmed/24106048 [cited 17 September 2018]

[96] Ohmi Y, Ise W, Harazono A, Takakura D, Fukuyama H, Baba Y, et al. Sialylation converts arthritogenic IgG into inhibitors of collagen-induced arthritis. Nature Communications. 2016; 7:11205. Available from: http://www.ncbi.nlm.nih.gov/pubmed/27046227 [cited 17 September 2018]

[97] Chen G, Wang Y, Qiu L, Qin X, Liu H, Wang X, et al. Human IgG Fc-glycosylation profiling reveals associations with age, sex, female sex hormones and thyroid cancer. Journal of Proteomics. 2012;**75**(10):2824-2834. Available from: http://www.ncbi.nlm.nih.gov/pubmed/22365975 [cited 17 September 2018]

[98] Engdahl C, Bondt A, Harre U, Raufer J, Pfeifle R, Camponeschi A, et al. Estrogen induces St6gal1 expression and increases IgG sialylation in mice and patients with rheumatoid arthritis: A potential explanation for the increased risk of rheumatoid arthritis in postmenopausal women. Arthritis Research & Therapy. 2018;**20**(1):84. Available from: http://www.ncbi.nlm.nih.gov/pubmed/29720252 [cited 17 September 2018]

[99] Stefano GB, Prevot V, Beauvillain JC, Fimiani C, Welters I, Cadet P, et al. Estradiol coupling to human monocyte nitric oxide release is dependent on intracellular calcium transients: Evidence for an estrogen surface receptor. The Journal of Immunology. 1999;**163**(7): 3758-3763. Available from: http://www.ncbi.nlm.nih.gov/pubmed/10490972 [cited 18 September 2018]

[100] Hess RA, Bunick D, Lee K-H, Bahr J, Taylor JA, Korach KS, et al. A role for oestrogens in the male reproductive system. Nature. 1997; **390**(6659):509-512. Available from: http://www.ncbi.nlm.nih.gov/pubmed/9393999 [cited 18 September 2018]

[101] Straub RH. The complex role of estrogens in inflammation. Endocrine

Reviews. 2007;**28**(5):521-574. Available from: http://www.ncbi.nlm.nih.gov/pubmed/17640948 [cited 12 September 2018]

[102] Trigunaite A, Dimo J, Jørgensen TN. Suppressive effects of androgens on the immune system. Cellular Immunology. 2015;**294**(2): 87-94. Available from: http://www.ncbi.nlm.nih.gov/pubmed/25708485 [cited 12 September 2018]

[103] Dubal DB, Zhu H, Yu J, Rau SW, Shughrue PJ, Merchenthaler I, et al. Estrogen receptor α, not β, is a critical link in estradiol-mediated protection against brain injury. Proceedings of the National Academy of Sciences. 2001; **98**(4):1952-1957. Available from: http://www.pnas.org/content/98/4/1952.long [cited 04 October 2018]

[104] Correale J, Arias M, Gilmore W. Steroid hormone regulation of cytokine secretion by proteolipid protein-specific CD4+ T cell clones isolated from multiple sclerosis patients and normal control subjects. The Journal of Immunology. 1998;**161**(7):3365-3374. Available from: http://www.ncbi.nlm.nih.gov/pubmed/9759853 [cited 17 September 2018]

[105] Hu SK, Mitcho YL, Rath NC. Effect of estradiol on interleukin 1 synthesis by macrophages. International Immunopharmacology. 1988;**10**(3): 247-252. Available from: http://www.ncbi.nlm.nih.gov/pubmed/3263330 [cited 17 September 2018]

[106] Murphy AJ, Guyre PM, Pioli PA. Estradiol suppresses NF-kappa B activation through coordinated regulation of let-7a and miR-125b in primary human macrophages. The Journal of Immunology. 2010;**184**(9): 5029-5037. Available from: http://www.ncbi.nlm.nih.gov/pubmed/20351193 [cited 21 September 2018]

[107] Capellino S, Montagna P, Villaggio B, Soldano S, Straub RH, Cutolo M. Hydroxylated estrogen metabolites influence the proliferation of cultured human monocytes: Possible role in synovial tissue hyperplasia. Clinical and Experimental Rheumatology. 2008;**26**(5): 903-909. Available from: http://www.ncbi.nlm.nih.gov/pubmed/19032826 [cited 18 September 2018]

[108] Yu F, Bender W. The mechanism of tamoxifen in breast cancer prevention. Breast Cancer Research. 2001;**3**(S1):A74. Available from: http://breast-cancer-research.biomedcentral.com/articles/10.1186/bcr404 [cited 08 October 2018]

[109] Ateka-Barrutia O, Nelson-Piercy C. Management of rheumatologic diseases in pregnancy. International Journal of Clinical Rheumatology. 2012;7:541-558. Available from: https://www.medscape.com/viewarticle/773344 [cited 14 September 2018]

[110] Lubahn DB, RRVHLKKLKPJA. Estrogen receptor α mediates estrogen's immune protection in autoimmune disease. Journal of Immunology Research. 2003;**171**:6936-6940. Available from: http://www.jimmunol.org/content/171/12/6936http://www.jimmunol.org/content/171/12/6936.full#ref-list-1 [cited 04 October 2018]

[111] Nakamura T, Imai Y, Matsumoto T, Sato S, Takeuchi K, Igarashi K, et al. Estrogen prevents bone loss via estrogen receptor alpha and induction of Fas ligand in osteoclasts. Cell. 2007;**130**(5): 811-823. Available from: http://www.ncbi.nlm.nih.gov/pubmed/17803905 [cited 27 September 2018]

[112] Josefsson E, Tarkowski A, Dahlin A-G, Crafoord F, Thuring I, Lundgren M, et al. Suppression of type II collagen-induced arthritis by the endogenous estrogen metabolite 2-methoxyestradiol. Arthritis & Rheumatism. January 1997; **40**(1):154-163. DOI: 10.1002/art.1780400120

[113] Lubahn DB. Estrogen receptor α mediates estrogen's immune protection in autoimmune disease. The Journal of Immunology. 2003;**171**:6936-6940

[114] Orellana C, Saevarsdottir S, Klareskog L, Karlson EW, Alfredsson L, Bengtsson C. Postmenopausal hormone therapy and the risk of rheumatoid arthritis: Results from the Swedish EIRA population-based case-control study. European Journal of Epidemiology. 2015;**30**(5):449-457. Available from: http://www.ncbi.nlm.nih.gov/pubmed/25762170 [cited 24 September 2018]

[115] Oliver JE, Silman AJ. Why are women predisposed to autoimmune rheumatic diseases? Arthritis Research & Therapy. 2009;**11**(5):252

[116] Hannaford PC, Kay CR, Hirsch S. Oral contraceptives and rheumatoid arthritis: New data from the Royal College of general practitioners' oral contraception study. Annals of the Rheumatic Diseases. 1990; **49**(10):744-746. Available from: http://www.ncbi.nlm.nih.gov/pubmed/2241261

[117] Reduction in incidence of rheumatoid arthritis associated with oral contraceptives. The Lancet. 1978; **311**(8064):569-571. Available from: https://linkinghub.elsevier.com/retrieve/pii/S014067367891022X [cited 11 September 2019]

[118] Orellana C, Saevarsdottir S, Klareskog L, Karlson EW, Alfredsson L, Bengtsson C. Oral contraceptives, breastfeeding and the risk of developing rheumatoid arthritis: Results from the Swedish EIRA study. Annals of the Rheumatic Diseases. 2017;**76**(11): 1845-1852. Available from: http://www.ncbi.nlm.nih.gov/pubmed/28818831 [cited 11 September 2019]

[119] Spector TD, Hochberg MC. The protective effect of the oral contraceptive pill on rheumatoid arthritis: An overview of the analytic epidemiological studies using meta-analysis. Journal of Clinical Epidemiology. 1990;**43**(11):1221-1230. Available from: http://www.ncbi.nlm.nih.gov/pubmed/2147033 [cited 11 September 2019]

[120] Qi S, Xin R, Guo W, Liu Y. Meta-analysis of oral contraceptives and rheumatoid arthritis risk in women. Therapeutics and Clinical Risk Management. 2014;**10**:915-923. Available from: http://www.ncbi.nlm.nih.gov/pubmed/25395857 [cited 21 September 2018]

[121] D'Elia HF, Larsen A, Mattsson L-A, Waltbrand E, Kvist G, Mellström D, et al. Influence of hormone replacement therapy on disease progression and bone mineral density in rheumatoid arthritis. The Journal of Rheumatology. 2003; **30**(7):1456-1463. Available from: http://www.ncbi.nlm.nih.gov/pubmed/12858441 [cited 17 September 2018]

[122] Hillard PA. Menstrual suppression: Current perspectives. International Journal of Women's Health. 2014;**6**: 631-637. Available from: http://www.ncbi.nlm.nih.gov/pubmed/25018654 [cited 21 September 2018]

[123] Cristofaro PA, Opal SM, Palardy JE, Parejo NA, Jhung J, Keith JC, et al. WAY-202196, a selective estrogen receptor-beta agonist, protects against death in experimental septic shock. Critical Care Medicine. 2006;**34**(8): 2188-2193. Available from: http://www.ncbi.nlm.nih.gov/pubmed/16755255 [cited 20 September 2018]

[124] Harris HA, Bruner-Tran KL, Zhang X, Osteen KG, Lyttle CR. A selective estrogen receptor-β agonist causes lesion regression in an experimentally induced model of endometriosis. Human Reproduction. 2005;**20**(4):936-941. Available from: http://www.ncbi.nlm.nih.gov/pubmed/15618247 [cited 20 September 2018]

[125] Cvoro A, Tatomer D, Tee M-K, Zogovic T, Harris HA, Leitman DC. Selective estrogen receptor-beta agonists repress transcription of proinflammatory genes. The Journal of Immunology. 2008;**180**(1):630-636. Available from: http://www.ncbi.nlm.nih.gov/pubmed/18097065 [cited 20 September 2018]

Chapter 3

Understanding the Mechanisms of Pain in Rheumatoid Arthritis

Kathryn Biddle and Nidhi Sofat

Abstract

Pain is a debilitating feature of rheumatoid arthritis (RA) and is often described by patients as their most important symptom. Rheumatoid arthritis pain has traditionally been attributed solely to joint inflammation, however despite the advent of increasingly effective disease modifying agents, patients continue to report pain at long term follow up. The cause for ongoing pain is multifactorial and includes joint damage and pain sensitisation. In this book chapter, we will describe the mechanisms underlying the distinct components of pain which are manifest in rheumatoid arthritis and discuss why a thorough assessment of pain is vital to target treatments appropriately.

Keywords: pain, rheumatoid arthritis, inflammation, pain sensitisation, nociceptors, rheumatology

1. Introduction

Rheumatoid arthritis (RA) is a systemic inflammatory disease with a prevalence of between 0.5 to 1% in different worldwide populations [1]. Inflammation predominantly affects the joints causing synovitis, pannus formation and if left untreated, joint destruction. Patients with RA classically present with tender and swollen joints, early morning joint stiffness and systemic symptoms such as fatigue. Severe pain is a particularly debilitating feature of RA that is commonly described as patients' most important symptom [2]. In addition to causing a significant impact on quality of life, studies have shown that RA pain is associated with psychological distress, impaired physical and social function and increased healthcare costs [3].

The pathogenesis of pain in RA is multifactorial. Traditionally, pain was entirely attributed to synovitis and consequent joint destruction. With the advent of increasingly effective disease modifying agents, joint inflammation has become a more treatable cause of pain and joint destruction is preventable. Indeed, the randomised controlled trials (RCTs) that supported the use of classical disease modifying anti-rheumatic drugs (DMARDs), showed statistically and clinically significant reduction in pain with treatment [4]. However, despite effective control of inflammation and disease remission, patients have continued to report troublesome pain at follow-up [5]. The same has been shown in patients taking biologic DMARDs [6]. This suggests that pain does not always fully resolve with the effective suppression of synovitis [7]. Observational studies have also highlighted the complex relationship between pain and inflammation in patients with RA. For example, large discrepancies between objective measures of inflammation such as acute-phase proteins and reported pain, have been shown in some patients with RA [8].

IntechOpen

Taken together, this evidence suggests that inflammation and joint destruction alone cannot account for the total pain manifesting in RA. Indeed, increasing evidence supports a role for aberrant pain processing, including peripheral and central pain sensitisation, in the pathogenesis of pain in RA. Throughout this book chapter, we will explore the different mechanisms underlying the perception of pain in patients with RA.

2. Inflammation in RA

RA is a pathologically heterogenous autoimmune condition. The disease can broadly be divided into sero-positive and sero-negative subtypes. In sero-positive patients, the presence of anti-citrullinated peptide antibodies (ACPAs), is associated with more severe joint damage and increased mortality [9]. In these patients, ACPAs bind to citrullinated autoantigens including fibrinogen, vimentin, collagen type 4 and α-enolase, resulting in the formation of immune complexes (ICs) [10]. ICs activate the complement system and trigger inflammatory cell infiltration within the synovium [11].

The pathology of RA is characterised by the activation of cells of both the innate and adaptive immune system within the synovial matrix. The innate immune response consists of macrophages, mast cells and dendritic cells. These cells produce inflammatory mediators including cytokines, chemokines, lipids, proteases and growth factors. These mediators attract neutrophils and activate cells of the adaptive immune system, such as T cells, B cells and plasma cells. The inflammatory cytokines produced during the innate immune response shape the subsequent activation of the adaptive immune system. For example, cytokines produced in the early phases of inflammation regulate the differentiation of naïve T helper cells into T helper cell subsets and the subsequent T cell response.

In RA, the inflammatory milieu within the synovium is characterised by complex cytokine and chemokine interactions. Cytokines including TNF-α and IL-6 appear to be particularly important, and biologic agents targeting these mediators are well-established treatments for RA [12].

Inflammation results in a catabolic state within the joint. One of the pathognomonic features of RA is the synovial pannus, a hypertrophied area of synovium with tissue destructive properties [13]. Within the pannus, synovial fibroblasts assume an inflammatory phenotype resulting in enhanced cartilage catabolism and synovial osteoclastogenesis [14]. Cytokine-mediated chondrocyte activation results in the stimulation of catabolic pathways. Enzymes including matrix metalloproteinases (MMPs) are activated to degrade the cartilage matrix [15]. Bone erosion is stimulated by the interaction between RANK-L on fibroblasts, T and B cells and its receptor RANK on dendritic cells, macrophages and pre-osteoclasts [16]. Ultimately, this process can result in cartilage and bone destruction and joint deformity.

Therapies that target inflammation such as conventional DMARDs and biologic therapies are effective at suppressing synovitis and reducing joint destruction. The treat-to-target approach is widely recommended for the management of RA. This strategy involves regular monitoring of disease activity, using validated scoring measures such as the DAS28, and escalation of treatment if a target is not reached. RCTs have found that this approach substantially improves disease activity, radiographic progression, quality of life and physical function [17]. These immunomodulatory agents have been shown to reduce pain, albeit not completely [18]. Throughout the next section of this chapter, we will discuss the inflammatory basis of pain in RA.

2.1 Pain and joint inflammation

Inflammation has long been accepted to cause pain. Indeed, pain was one of the cardinal features of inflammation, as defined by Celsus in the first century [19]. Pain secondary to inflammation can be classified into acute or chronic pain. The neurotransmission of acute pain signals in response to noxious stimulation involves the activation of a specialised subset of sensory neurons called nociceptors. Nociceptors innervate peripheral tissues, including joints, and transmit painful stimuli to the dorsal root ganglion (DRG). There are many subsets of nociceptors, each responding to different types of noxious stimuli. Aδ and C fibres are the two main types of primary afferent nociceptors [20]. Whilst both Aδ and C fibres are found in superficial organs, such as the skin, C-fibres generally supply deeper structures such as joints [20]. C-fibres are activated by thermal, chemical or mechanical stimulation, resulting in poorly localised, dull pain sensation [20].

The activation of nociceptors involves the stimulation of ligand-gated and voltage-gated ion channels including transient receptor potential cation channel, subfamily A, member 1 (TRPV1), transient receptor potential cation channel, subfamily A, member 1 (TRPA1), $Na_v1.7$, $Na_v1.8$, and $Na_v1.9$ channels, which are expressed on peripheral nerve terminals [21]. Activation of these channels results in the stimulation of intracellular signalling pathways and the transmission of acute pain signals [21]. In the longer term, chronic inflammation results in long lasting changes in nociceptor signalling resulting in peripheral pain sensitisation, a phenomenon that we will discuss later in this chapter.

2.2 Synovial joint structures and pain

Arthritic pain is thought to be mediated by nociceptors that innervate the synovium and subchondral bone. In contrast, under physiological conditions, cartilage is an aneural and avascular tissue. This is illustrated in **Figure 1**.

In RA, chronic inflammation is thought to result in structural and functional changes in the peripheral innervation of joints. This has been shown in animal

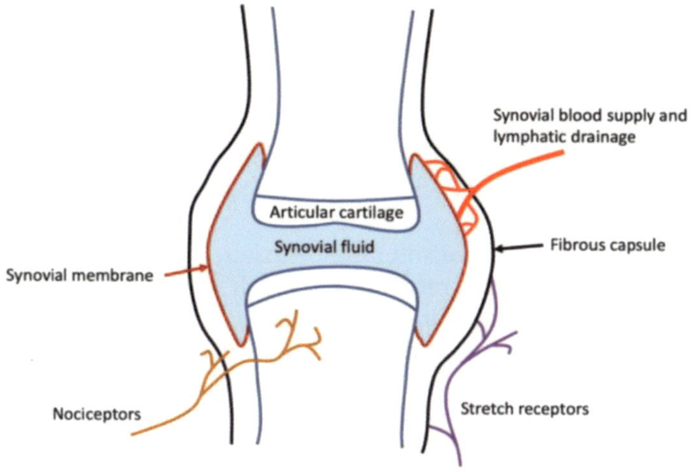

Figure 1.
Diagram of a synovial joint. A synovial joint consists of two articulating cartilage surfaces surrounded by a synovial membrane. Synovial fluid fills the synovium. Under physiological conditions, cartilage is avascular and aneural. Nociceptors innervating the synovium and subchondral bone are responsible for arthritic pain. In contrast, stretch receptors, innervating the fibrous capsule are responsible for proprioception.

models where chronic synovitis results in increased innervation of the synovium and increased spontaneous and mechanical-induced firing of articular primary afferents [22, 23].

2.3 Nociceptor pathways

Nociceptor pathways mediating acute pain perception in response to inflammation are well defined. In the periphery, local immune cells release inflammatory mediators, such as cytokines, that act on the peripheral nerve terminals of nociceptor neurons. This activates the nociceptors to transmit signals via the DRG through the spinothalamic tract to the higher cortical centres, resulting in the perception of pain. It is also well accepted that inflammation can result in heightened nociceptor sensitivity to both noxious and innocuous stimuli. In this case, the activation of nociceptors by inflammatory mediators triggers intracellular signalling cascades that reduce the threshold for nociceptor neurons to fire action potentials [21]. This results in heightened pain sensitivity which can manifest as allodynia; the sensation of pain arising from a non-painful stimulus, or hyperalgesia; a heightened sensation of pain in response to painful stimulation. Throughout the next section of this chapter, we will discuss the inflammatory mediators that stimulate nociceptor activation and sensitisation in RA.

2.4 Pain and innate immunity

Cells of the innate immune system, including neutrophils, mast cells and macrophages, release noxious inflammatory mediators and have been shown to stimulate pain and pain sensitisation in a wide range of models and systems. For example, in mouse models of carrageenan-induced inflammatory pain, neutrophils migrate to tissues and sustain pain through the production of cytokines and prostaglandin E2 [24]. In incisional wound injury, macrophages (CD11b + myeloid cells) have been shown to mediate acute pain and pain sensitisation [25]. Mast cell degranulation activates nociceptor firing acutely and may also contribute to pathology of chronic pain and mast cells have been shown accumulate in chronic inflammatory conditions such as complex regional pain syndrome [26, 27]. Throughout the next part of the chapter, we will discuss the noxious inflammatory mediators that are released by innate immune cells.

2.5 Lipid mediators of pain

Pro-inflammatory lipids include cyclooxygenase (COX) dependent molecules such as prostanoids (prostaglandins, prostacyclins and thromboxanes). COX-dependent molecules are well known to cause pain and pain sensitisation and inhibition of the COX enzyme, using non-steroidal anti-inflammatory drugs (NSAIDs), is used for the suppression of pain and inflammation. Indeed, NSAIDs are potent analgesic and anti-inflammatory medications which are effective for the treatment of acute inflammatory pain including synovitis [28].

Studies have investigated the mechanism of action underlying the noxious effect of prostaglandins. Prostaglandin E2 (PGE2) has been shown to activate nociceptors through the binding of EP1-EP4 receptors. This stimulates pain and pain sensitisation via multiple mechanisms. PGE2 stimulates proximal ion channels in nociceptive neurons. This sensitises the neurons to painful stimuli [29]. PGE2 activates more persistent pain sensitisation via PKA and PKC-mediated activation of NFκB in the dorsal root ganglion neurons [30].

Many other classes of pro-inflammatory lipids are thought to be involved in the activation of nociceptor activity. For example, lysophosphatidic acid and sphingosine-1-phosphate are produced during inflammation and have been shown to activate nociceptors leading to increased TRPV1 activity [31]. Leukotrienes may also have an noxious effect and the injection of leukotriene B4 has been shown to activate C and Aδ-fibres in rat models and induce hyperalgesia in humans [21, 32].

More recent work has also demonstrated a role for anti-inflammatory and pro-resolving lipids in the silencing of pain. For example, pro-resolving lipids, including lipoxins, resolvins and protectins have generally been shown to have analgesic effects [33]. Further work is required to characterise the underlying molecular pathways but these mediators may represent targets for the future treatment of pain [33].

2.6 Neurotransmitters and pain

Innate immune cells release neurotransmitters capable of modulating pain transmission. For example, mast cells contain histamine and serotonin that are released on degranulation. Histamine triggers pain sensitisation through the activation of H1 and H2 receptors expressed on nociceptors [34]. This results in increased expression of Nav1.8 channels and increased sensitivity to noxious stimuli [34, 35].

2.7 Cytokines and pain

Inflammatory cytokines represent another important class of molecules that stimulate nociceptors and activate pain sensitisation. IL-1β was the first cytokine to be described as hyperalgesic [36]. This finding was seminal in the field of neuro-immunology and represented early evidence for the cross-talk between the immune system and pain sensitisation. Cytokines have now been found to play important roles in pain modulation in most painful conditions, including RA. Notably, pro-inflammatory cytokines including IL-1β, IL-6, TNF-α, IL-17A and IL-5, have all been shown to active nociceptors directly [21].

IL-1β sensitises nociceptors through different intra-cellular signalling pathways. Firstly, IL-1β activates the p38 MAPK-mediated phosphorylation of Nav1.8 sodium channels resulting in increased action potential generation and an associated mechanical and thermal hyperalgesia [37]. Secondly, the activation of IL-1R1 by IL1-β, has also been shown to result in increased TRPV1 expression on nociceptors, resulting in thermal pain sensitisation in animal models [38].

IL-6 stimulates pain sensitisation directly and indirectly. Directly, IL-6 activates nociceptors via the signal transducer gp 130 leading to increased TRPV1 and TRPA1 expression [39]. Indirectly, IL-6 activates nociceptors via the production of prostaglandins [39]. TNF-α also induces pain sensitisation via TRPA1 and TRPV1, however TNF-α mediated inflammatory pain appears to be dependent on prostaglandins [40]. Indeed, COX-2 inhibitors have been shown to inhibit TNF-α induced capsaicin responsiveness in cultured nociceptors [41]. TNF-α also modulates nociceptor sensitivity through the activation of p38 MAPK mediated phosphorylation of Nav.18 and Nav1.9 sodium channels [42].

Increasing work suggests a role for IL-17 in pain sensitisation. Indeed, many painful autoimmune diseases, such as RA and psoriasis, are characterised by a Th17 immune response. IL-17A has been shown to be broadly expressed by nociceptors and IL-17 has been demonstrated to induce a rapid increase in neuronal excitability [43]. In animal models of RA, IL-17 has been shown to induce hyperalgesia, through a mechanism dependent on the amplification of TNF-α, IL-1B, CXCL-1, endothelin 1 and prostaglandins [44].

In summary, IL-1β, IL-6, TNF-α and IL-17 stimulate pain and pain sensitisation through the synthesis of prostaglandins and/or the activation of sodium or TRP channels. The different cytokines appear to act via different intracellular signalling pathways, however it remains unclear whether different immune responses (e.g. Th1, Th2 or Th17) induce different pain characteristics through the activation of specific nociceptors and pain receptors.

2.8 Immune derived growth factors in pain

Innervation by nociceptors is a dynamic process affected by neurotrophic factors. These factors are often upregulated in response to inflammation or tissue injury and are important to restore the density of innervation post-injury [21]. If there is inappropriate or excessive release of neurotrophic factors, heightened pain sensitivity can occur [21]. Nerve growth factor (NGF) is an important neurotrophic factor that is secreted by innate immune cells during the acute phase of inflammation. NGF activates the receptor TrkA on nociceptors, stimulating the P13K/Src kinase pathway and the phosphorylation of TRPV1 and its translocation into the cell membrane [45]. This results in the rapid sensitisation of nociceptors in response to stimulation by NGF. In the longer term, NGF has been shown to stimulate axonal terminal sprouting, contributing to increased pain sensitivity [46].

2.9 A role for ACPAs in pain in RA

It is well established that arthralgia can precede overt joint inflammation and that joint pain is often one of the first symptoms of emerging RA. The mechanism underlying arthralgia preceding inflammation remains unclear but a role for ACPAs has been suggested. Observational studies have shown that ACPAs frequently occur in the preclinical phase of disease and can be detected months to years prior

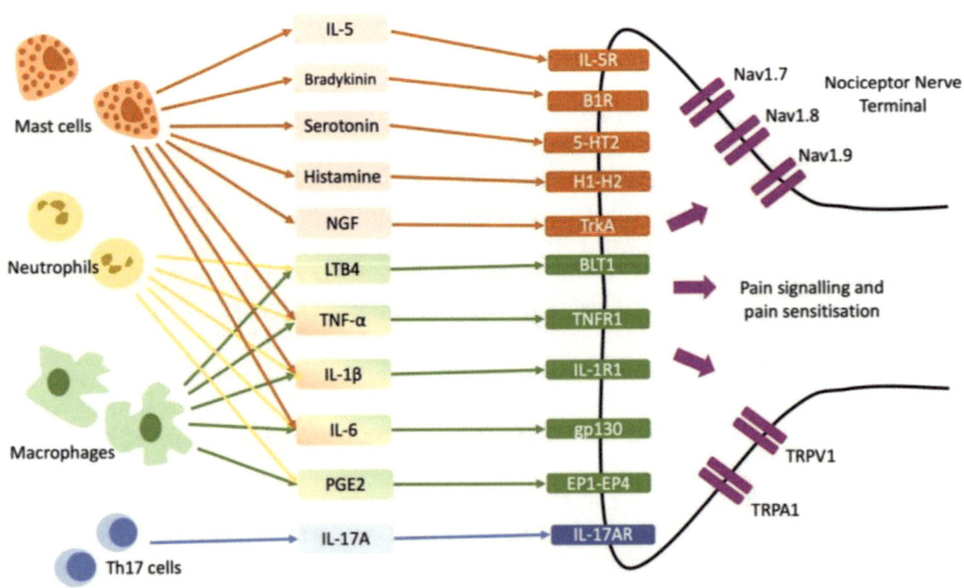

Figure 2.
Inflammatory mediators and pain. ***Figure 2*** *Summarises the inflammatory mediators that have been shown to activate and sensitise nociceptors[21]. As illustrated, innate and adaptive immune cells release inflammatory mediators that act on their respective receptors to activate nociceptors and sensitise pain signalling through Nav and TRP channels.*

to diagnosis [47]. Experimental studies have raised the possibility that ACPAs can induce pain via a pathway independent of joint inflammation. In one study, mice injected with human or murine ACPAs developed increased pain sensitivity, despite no signs of joint inflammation. In this study, ACPAs were shown to bind to osteoclasts in the bone marrow, and induce CXCL1/2 expression and release. Intra-articular injection of CXCL1/2 was shown to evoke pain-like behaviour and this was inhibited by an IL-8 inhibitor, reparixin [48]. Further work is required to confirm this hypothesis. If correct, it could alter the management of ACPA positive arthralgia and offer new therapeutic targets in the management of early RA.

In summary, inflammation is a well-accepted cause of pain in RA and many inflammatory mediators have been shown to stimulate nociceptor activation and sensitisation, as summarised in **Figure 2**.

Despite the important role for inflammation in pain in RA, the extent of inflammation does not always correlate with the severity of total pain reported RA patients. Indeed, observational studies have shown that changes in inflammation account for only 40% of changes in pain in RA patients [49]. Furthermore, factors associated with the degree of inflammation such as serology, acute phase response and joint damage correlate poorly with pain prognosis in RA patients [7]. Moreover, in common with other chronic pain conditions, psychosocial factors and female gender predict pain prognosis more accurately than the severity of inflammation [7]. Therefore, additional mechanisms must be responsible for the pain experienced in RA. These mechanisms include joint damage and aberrant pain sensitisation.

3. Joint damage and pain

The contribution of structural joint changes to the total pain in RA is controversial. In patients with advanced RA, erosions and joint space narrowing are associated with disability and make a small but significant contribution to total reported pain [50]. Moreover, patients with advanced disease show an improvement in pain following joint replacement surgery [51]. However, as more effective disease modifying protocols have been developed, structural joint damage in RA has decreased and corresponding rates of orthopaedic surgery have declined [52]. The prevention of joint damage has produced superior pain outcomes but it is not clear how much of this can be attributed to the prevention of structural damage versus the suppression of inflammation or prevention of pain sensitisation. In recent studies, radiographically assessed joint damage appears to make a small contribution to pain in RA patients [53]. However, some of this pain may be explained by coincident osteoarthritis (OA), which occurs in a similar demographic of patients.

The correlation between joint damage and pain severity appears weak, although investigation on this subject has primarily occurred in patients with OA and relatively little data exists for patients with RA. In OA, structural joint changes do not correlate well with joint pain [54]. The severity of radiographic OA has been shown to explain <20% of the variance in pain intensity [54]. Furthermore, post-joint replacement, many patients continue to report pain. 10% of patients post-total hip replacement (THR) and 20% post-total knee replacement (TKR) report unfavourable long term pain outcomes [55]. This suggests that structural joint damage alone cannot explain the total pain experienced in OA. Like in RA, central pain sensitisation has been proposed to explain the pain not accounted for by joint destruction [56].

4. Central pain sensitisation and RA

Processing by the central nervous system (CNS) can affect pain reporting, sensitivity, intensity and pain characteristics [57]. Aberrant pain processing can result in central pain sensitisation; an amplified response of the central nervous system to peripheral nociceptive input [58]. The term central sensitisation was coined in 1989 by Woolf and colleagues based on work in the rat model showing hyperexcitability of spinal cord neurons in response to peripheral tissue injury [58]. Physiologically, central sensitisation represents a state of hyperexcitability of spinal and supra-spinal structures due to amplified neuronal signalling involving enhanced synaptic and neurotransmitter activities [59].

An increasing abundance of evidence supports the role for central pain sensitisation in RA and an understanding of central sensitisation is important to optimise patient treatment. Clinically, pain secondary to an inflammatory flare must be differentiated from pain secondary to central sensitisation as they require vastly different management approaches. Throughout the next part of this chapter, we will discuss the molecular basis of pain transmission from the periphery to the CNS, clinical evidence supporting a role for pain sensitisation in RA and some proposed mechanisms for pain sensitisation in the DRG and in the cerebral cortex.

4.1 Molecular basis of pain sensitisation

As discussed previously, A-δ and C nociceptive neurons are activated by inflammatory mediators in the periphery. These fibres converge at the DRG, along with non-noxious A-β fibres. Following activation, nociceptor fibres release substance P (SP), calcitonin gene-related peptide (CGRP), glutamate, aspartate and NGF at the afferent nerve endings into the synaptic cleft [60]. These neurotransmitters activate their corresponding receptors on post-synaptic neurons. Activation of post-synaptic receptors results in intracellular signalling changes. For example, activation of NMDA receptors results in increased membrane permeability, intracellular entry of calcium, activation of protein kinases and the expression of c-fos [61]. These signalling changes result in the hyperexcitability of the secondary neurons and amplification of the peripheral noxious stimulus. Post-synaptic neurons ascend in the spinothalamic tract to the thalamus, hypothalamus, limbic system and the somatosensory cortex [61]. These signalling pathways are summarised in **Figure 3**.

Animal models of RA have been used to investigate the molecular mechanisms underlying spinal pain sensitisation. In these models, molecular changes have been shown to occur in the DRG, spinal neurons and spinoreticular neurons. For example, in complete Freund's adjuvant (CFA) induced arthritis models, increased expression of SP, CGRP, NPY, c-fos, TRPV1, P2X3 and Trk-A receptors in the DRG have been demonstrated [62]. These changes are thought to result in hyperexcitability of spinal neurons and enhanced sensitivity to nociceptor signalling.

4.2 Clinical evidence for a role of pain sensitisation in RA

Patients with RA show widespread reductions in pain threshold and increased pain sensitivity, not only over inflamed joints but at distant, non-articular sites [62]. Evidence to support this has come from clinical studies using techniques such as quantitative sensory testing (QST). This technique involves the application of stimuli under standardised testing protocols and the quantification of the participants sensory experience. QST employs different tools for the assessment of the perception of vibration, touch, proprioception, pinprick or blunt pressure

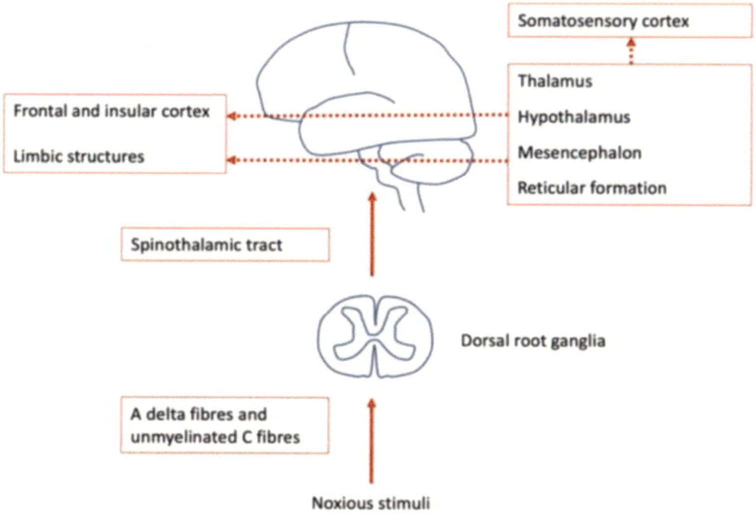

Figure 3.
A simplified diagram of pain signalling pathways. As illustrated, noxious stimulation activates A-δ and C fibres in the periphery. These fibres converge at the DRG and activate post-synaptic neurons that ascend to higher cortical centres via the spinothalamic tract.

sensitivity. RA patients have a lower pain threshold than healthy controls with QST [63]. Furthermore, sensitisation has been shown to affect a wide range of sensory modalities, including thermal and mechanical stimulation.

Studies have demonstrated that pain thresholds vary substantially between patients with RA. Multiple factors have been shown to correlate with differences in pain threshold. Importantly, these include high tender joint count and prolonged disease duration [64]. This suggests that the persistence of nociceptive stimulation results in long-term changes in pain processing resulting in central pain sensitisation. Other factors that have been shown to influence pain threshold include sleep quality, psychosocial factors and analgesic use [65].

Repetitive sensory stimulation, also known as temporal summation, is another experimental model that has been used to investigate central sensitisation in RA. Temporal summation occurs when the time between stimuli is short enough to prevent the dissipation of postsynaptic action potentials before re-activation [66]. This results in a higher membrane potential, increasing the probability that further stimulation will result in post-synaptic activation. In healthy controls, repetitive stimulation results in the reduction of pressure pain thresholds [62]. Studies have shown that this response is augmented in RA patients [67]. This has also been demonstrated electrophysiologically through the measurement of action potentials in response to repetitive stimulation. In healthy controls, there is an increase in the amplitude of action potential evoked from repetitive stimulation using noxious stimulation. This response is amplified in RA patients and has been shown to correlate with disease activity scores and high tender joint counts [68].

4.3 Neuropathic pain in RA

In addition to measuring pain thresholds, pain characteristics can be analysed to assess the possible contribution of pain sensitisation to overall pain experience. Specifically, pain questionnaires are commonly used to detect the presence of neuropathic-sounding pain. Neuropathic pain is the perception of pain in the absence of nociceptive input or peripheral tissue damage and is caused by pathology of the peripheral or central nerves. A classic example of neuropathic pain is sciatica. This pain has distinct characteristics such as burning, radiation, shooting, tingling and sensitivity to non-painful stimuli (i.e. allodynia). RA can be associated with neuropathic pain through several mechanisms including compression neuropathy (e.g. carpal tunnel syndrome), co-morbidities (e.g. diabetes), vasculitis (resulting in mononeuritis multiplex) or drug therapies (e.g. gold or leflunomide). Nevertheless, emerging evidence suggests that RA itself can result in neuropathic pain through the induction of aberrant pain processing.

The painDETECT questionnaire enables the classification of pain into likely, possibly or unlikely to be of neuropathic origin. Patients with RA often describe pain with neuropathic features and painDETECT questionnaires can yield between 5 to 20% fulfilling criteria for "likely neuropathic pain" [62]. A significant proportion of these patients have no underlying evidence of neuropathy. One study demonstrated that only 33% of RA patients fulfilling clinical criteria for neuropathic pain had clinical evidence of neuropathy [69]. Of the remaining patients, 57% were shown to have subclinical or axonal neuropathy [70]. This left a significant number of patients with RA who reported neuropathic-sounding pain in the absence of objective nerve injury. It has been suggested that this pain occurs secondary to pain sensitisation however, this has not been proven. Nevertheless, neuropathic-sounding pain is an important clinical feature as it predicts inferior pain outcomes. Indeed, a positive correlation between VAS pain scores and painDETECT scores has been demonstrated and patients with probable or likely neuropathic pain have been shown to report significantly higher VAS scores than patients without neuropathic-sounding pain [71].

Although the painDETECT questionnaire is a useful tool for characterising pain, care must be taken to interpret results based only on questionnaires. Furthermore, confounding effects with pain severity may affect interpretation. Patients with fibromyalgia demonstrate high painDETECT scores, although evidence of pathology in the peripheral or central nervous system has been difficult to demonstrate. This raises the question of whether painDETECT scores identify pain with similar features to neuropathic pain rather than neuronal pathology itself. Further work is required to fully understand the significance of neuropathic sounding pain in RA.

4.4 Fibromyalgia-RA

The association between fibromyalgia and RA sheds light on the complex relationship between inflammation, pain and central pain sensitisation. Fibromyalgia (FM) is the prototypical central pain sensitivity syndrome. Clinically, FM is characterised by chronic widespread pain, sleep disturbance and impaired cognition [72]. Observational studies have shown that the prevalence of fibromyalgia in RA patients is much higher than in the general population with estimated prevalence of 18-24%, compared to 2-4% in non-RA cohorts [73, 74].

Two groups of fibromyalgia (FM) have been characterised. Patients with "primary" FM report pain in the absence of identifiable nociceptive input [72]. These patients generally report regional pain syndromes that progress to widespread pain phenotypes with time. "Secondary" FM occurs when aberrant centralised pain processing occurs in the context of identifiable nociceptive input, for example in inflammatory arthritis [72]. It is not yet clear whether these conditions represent the same or different diseases.

The co-existence of FM in RA patients is associated with increased pain scores, a poorer quality of life and worse patient-reported outcomes. In a meta-analysis of 18 studies, RA patients with co-morbid FM had significantly higher pooled DAS28 scores than those without FM [73]. When studies reported individual components of the DAS28, patients with co-existent FM had significantly higher tender joint counts and higher patient global assessment scores than those without FM [73]. Objective measurements including swollen joints and inflammatory markers were not significantly different between RA patients with and without FM [73]. Other scoring systems including the simplified disease activity index (SDAI) and the clinical disease activity index (CDAI) were also higher in RA patients with comorbid FM [75]. A large study of 11,866 RA patients reported that those with comorbid FM had increased pain, poorer quality of life and greater functional limitation [76].

The recognition of FM in RA patients is important for multiple reasons. Firstly, both RA and FM commonly present with pain and fatigue. Differentiation of the conditions and diagnosis of co-morbidity is vital for patient management as different treatment approaches are required. In FM-RA patients, characterisation of the pain is imperative to manage patients appropriately. For example, inflammatory flares must be differentiated from painful flares secondary to FM. Secondly; recognition of patients with secondary FM offers an important insight into the pathogenesis of pain centralisation which is currently poorly understood. Nevertheless, caution should be used when interpreting the association between inflammatory arthritis and FM as the FM diagnostic tools have not been validated in RA. Furthermore, confounding factors including female sex and mental health problems are more prevalent in both FM and RA.

4.5 Central mechanisms of pain sensitisation

Central pain sensitisation is thought to occur at both spinal and supraspinal levels [62]. At the level of the DRG, spinal hyperexcitability occurs secondary to ongoing nociceptive input and pain transmission can be modified by inhibitory or facilitating neurones that can be modulated by descending signals from supraspinal levels [72]. Spinal pain facilitation is thought to be responsible for the spread of mechanical allodynia beyond the innervated field of cutaneous neurons. This has been shown in models using the intradermal injection of capsaicin [77]. Both ipsilateral and contralateral pain facilitation is thought to occur secondary to chronic inflammation and in RA patients, enhanced responses to noxious stimulation occurs at sites distal from inflamed joints [78]. Pain sensitisation is also thought to occur at supraspinal levels and brain imaging has demonstrated changes in cerebral activation secondary to chronic pain. Throughout the next section of the chapter, we will discuss the evidence of supraspinal pain sensitisation in RA.

4.6 Brain neuroimaging and pain

Imaging studies have attempted to characterise the neuronal circuitry resulting in cerebral sensitisation in RA. Structural MRI studies have shown increased grey matter density in the basal ganglia of RA patients compared to controls. This area is involved in both motor function and in pain processing [79]. Functional imaging has been used to investigate neuronal activation in response to pain. Functional MRI (fMRI) studies have demonstrated differences in resting state functional connectivity between RA patients and controls. In RA patients, there is increased connectivity between frontal midline regions that are implicated in pain processing, including the supplementary motor area and the mid-cingulate cortex, to sensorimotor regions [80]. Moreover, in RA patients, increased EEG activity has been reported in response to repetitive painful stimuli [81]. These studies suggest that aberrant pain cerebral pain processing may occur in RA and therefore, may result in augmented pain responses.

A further level of complexity is introduced when the biopsychosocial model of pain is considered. This suggests that cognitive and emotional processes are also critical contributors to the overall perception of pain. Indeed, the transmission of nociceptive information is influenced by multiple higher-level factors, such as mood, attention and cognitive factors, to form the resulting pain experience [82]. Mood is a particularly important cognitive factor in RA and meta-analysis has revealed that 16.8% of patients with RA meet the criteria for a major depressive episode [83].

In RA patients, depressive symptoms have been found to correlate significantly with tender joint count [84]. The medial prefrontal cortex has been suggested to play an important role in mediating the relationship between pain severity and depressive symptoms. Evidence has demonstrated an association between depressive scores (measured using the Becks depression index), tender joint count and MPFC activation during provoked joint pain. In the same study, MPFC activation co-varied significantly with limbic activation, an area involved in affective processing. This led the authors to suggest that the MPFC engages areas important for self-relevant processing to mediate the relationship between pain and affective symptoms [84]. In summary, pain processing by higher brain centres affects pain perception and the affective response to pain in RA. Although we are beginning to shed light on higher processing using functional imaging studies, more work is required to fully appreciate the complexities of central pain processing in RA.

5. Management of pain in RA

The cornerstone of RA treatment is the suppression of inflammation using the treat to target approach. However, disease remission will not lead to the complete resolution of pain in all patients and a multi-modal approach to pain management is very important. This approach has been recommended by rheumatology associations. For example, EULAR have recommended a patient centred approach to pain management where a biopsychosocial framework should be adopted [85]. Specifically, clinicians should differentiate between local and generalised pain and should be guided by patient needs, preferences, pain characteristics, inflammation and psychological factors. Treatments should include education, psychical therapies, orthotics, psychosocial interventions, sleep hygiene, pharmacological and joint-specific treatment options. Throughout this section of the review, we will discuss the different facets of pain management.

5.1 Pharmacological therapies

Pharmacological treatments include analgesic agents and immunomodulatory medications. Many analgesic agents are used in the management of RA pain although their use is rarely supported by high-quality RCTs [62]. Commonly used analgesic medications include paracetamol, NSAIDs, opioids and tricyclic anti-depressants. Optimal pain management should involve the characterisation of pain phenotype, in particular, differentiation of peripheral and central pain mechanisms. Pain phenotype could alter the choice of analgesic agent. For example, NSAIDs have been shown to reduce inflammatory pain in RA but not central pain in FM [86]. More work is required to define optimal analgesic use in different subsets of RA patients.

The cornerstone of RA management is the suppression of inflammation. Medications that reduce synovial inflammation are well known to reduce pain in RA patients. Immunomodulatory medications used in RA include glucocorticoids, conventional synthetic DMARDs and biologic DMARDs. Glucocorticoids are commonly used to treat acute inflammatory flares and have been shown to provide significant pain relief [87]. Extensive evidence supports the efficacy of traditional DMARDs, including methotrexate, sulfasalazine and leflunomide, in reducing joint pain. The analgesic effect of cDMARDs parallels the suppression over a time course of weeks to months [62]. Combination therapy has been shown to be superior than monotherapy and the addition of a biologic agent has been shown to reduce pain even further [88, 89]. Nevertheless, pain improvement may plateau despite effective suppression of inflammation and studies have shown that this plateau is worse that the UK mean [7]. Persisting pain may result from centrally mediated pain hypersensitivity and may respond better to neuropathic agents or non-pharmacological treatments including education, exercise and cognitive behavioural therapy (CBT) than those treatments focusing on management on nociceptive triggers alone.

5.2 Neuropathic agents

Neuromodulatory medications used for the treatment of neuropathic pain include antidepressants such as tricyclic antidepressants (e.g. amitriptyline) and serotonin-noradrenaline re-uptake inhibitors (e.g. duloxetine) or anti-convulsants, e.g., pregabalin or gabapentin [90]. The clinical efficacy of these medications well well-established in conditions including neuropathic pain and generalised pain sensitisation syndromes such as fibromyalgia [91, 92]. Neuropathic agents are sometimes used for the treatment of pain in RA however evidence from high quality RCTs is lacking [93]. However, in other localised pain conditions such as hand OA, pregabalin has been shown to improve pain and function [94]. Further work is required to establish the role for neuropathic medications in RA patients.

5.3 Psychosocial therapies

Psychological pain management programmes, including cognitive behavioural approaches and mindfulness, have an important role in the management of chronic pain. An abundance of evidence supports the efficacy of psychosocial approaches to pain management in chronic pain conditions [95]. In RA, CBT has the best evidence base for the management of pain with multiple meta-analyses confirming efficacy [96, 97]. In addition to benefiting pain symptoms, CBT has been shown to improve other symptoms including fatigue in RA patients [98]. Psychosocial therapy may be most efficacious when offered early in the disease course however further work is required to determine which subset of patients should be offered psychosocial therapies and at which time-point in their illness [99].

5.4 Exercise based therapies

Exercise based therapies have an important role in the management of RA. Evidence has shown that resistance exercises decrease disability and functional impairment [100]. Furthermore, a meta-analysis of five studies revealed that resistance exercises resulted in a trend towards a small positive effect on VAS pain [100].

6. Conclusion

In conclusion, pain remains a significant problem for many patients with RA and is associated with psychological distress, fatigue and reduced quality of life.

In RA patients, pain results from a combination of joint inflammation, structural joint changes and pain sensitisation. In order to treat patients effectively, it is vital to differentiate between different types of pain, as each type should be targeted differently. Effective pain management approaches using a multimodal approach are vital to increase patient well-being, functioning and to reduce individual and societal costs [85].

List of abbreviations

ACPA	anti-citrullinated peptide antibodies
CBT	cognitive behavioural therapy
CDAI	clinical disease activity index
CGRP	calcitonin gene-related peptide
CNS	central nervous system
COX	cyclooxygenase
CXCL	chemokine (C-X-C motif) ligand
DAS	disease activity score
DMARDs	disease modifying anti-rheumatic drugs
DRG	dorsal root ganglia
EEG	electroencephalogram
EULAR	European league against rheumatism
FM	fibromyalgia
fMRI	functional magnetic resonance imaging
IC	immune complexes
IL	interleukin
MAPK	mitogen activated protein kinase
MMP	matrix mellatoproteinase
MPFC	medial prefrontal cortex
MRI	magnetic resonance imaging
NFκB	nuclear factor kappa-light-chain-enhancer of activated B cells
NGF	nerve growth factor
NPY	neuropeptide Y
NSAIDs	non-steroidal anti-inflammatory drugs
OA	osteoarthritis
PI3K	phosphoinositide 3-kinases
PGE	prostaglandin E
PK	protein kinase
QST	quantitative sensory testing
RA	rheumatoid arthritis
RANK	receptor activator of nuclear factor kappa beta
RANK-L	receptor activator of nuclear factor kappa beta ligand
RCT	randomised control trials
SDAI	simple disease activity index
SP	substance P
THR	total hip replacement
TKR	total knee replacement
TNF	tumour necrosis factor
TrkA	tropomyosin receptor kinase A
TRPA1	transient receptor potential cation channel, subfamily A, member 1
TRPV1	transient receptor potential cation channel subfamily V member 1
VAS	visual analogue scale

Author details

Kathryn Biddle and Nidhi Sofat*
Musculoskeletal Research Group, Institute for Infection and Immunity, St George's, University of London, London, United Kingdom

*Address all correspondence to: nsofat@sgul.ac.uk

References

[1] Y. Alamanos, P. V. Voulgari, and A. A. Drosos, "Incidence and Prevalence of Rheumatoid Arthritis, Based on the 1987 American College of Rheumatology Criteria: A Systematic Review," Semin. Arthritis Rheum., 2006.

[2] T. Heiberg and T. K. Kvien, "Preferences for improved health examined in 1,024 patients with rheumatoid arthritis: Pain has highest priority," Arthritis Rheum., 2002.

[3] G. da Rocha Castelar Pinheiro, R. K. Khandker, R. Sato, A. Rose, and J. Piercy, "Impact of rheumatoid arthritis on quality of life, work productivity and resource utilisation: An observational, cross-sectional study in Brazil," Clin. Exp. Rheumatol., 2013.

[4] H. J. Williams et al., "Comparison of low-dose oral pulse methotrexate and placebo in the treatment of rheumatoid arthritis. A Controlled Clinical Trial," Arthritis Rheum., 1985.

[5] R. Altawil, S. Saevarsdottir, S. Wedrén, L. Alfredsson, L. Klareskog, and J. Lampa, "Remaining Pain in Early Rheumatoid Arthritis Patients Treated With Methotrexate," Arthritis Care Res., 2016.

[6] D. F. McWilliams and D. A. Walsh, "Factors predicting pain and early discontinuation of tumour necrosis factor-α-inhibitors in people with rheumatoid arthritis: Results from the British society for rheumatology biologics register," BMC Musculoskelet. Disord., 2016.

[7] D. F. McWilliams, W. Zhang, J. S. Mansell, P. D. W. Kiely, A. Young, and D. A. Walsh, "Predictors of change in bodily pain in early rheumatoid arthritis: An inception cohort study," Arthritis Care Res., 2012.

[8] S. J. Bartlett et al., "Identifying core domains to assess flare in rheumatoid arthritis: An OMERACT international patient and provider combined Delphi consensus," Ann. Rheum. Dis., 2012.

[9] D. Aletaha, F. Alasti, and J. S. Smolen, "Rheumatoid factor, not antibodies against citrullinated proteins, is associated with baseline disease activity in rheumatoid arthritis clinical trials," Arthritis Res. Ther., 2015.

[10] L. Klareskog, K. Lundberg, and V. Malmström, "Autoimmunity in Rheumatoid Arthritis: Citrulline Immunity and Beyond," in Advances in Immunology, 2013.

[11] X. Zhao et al., "Circulating immune complexes contain citrullinated fibrinogen in rheumatoid arthritis," Arthritis Res. Ther., 2008.

[12] M. Feldmann and S. R. N. Maini, "Role of cytokines in rheumatoid arthritis: An education in pathophysiology and therapeutics," Immunological Reviews. 2008.

[13] C. M. Weyand and J. J. Goronzy, "Immunometabolism in early and late stages of rheumatoid arthritis," Nature Reviews Rheumatology. 2017.

[14] I. B. McInnes and G. Schett, "The pathogenesis of rheumatoid arthritis.," The New England journal of medicine. 2011.

[15] J. Martel-Pelletier, D. J. Welsch, and J. P. Pelletier, "Metalloproteases and inhibitors in arthritic diseases," Best Pract. Res. Clin. Rheumatol., 2001.

[16] K. Redlich et al., "Osteoclasts are essential for TNF-α-mediated joint destruction," J. Clin. Invest., 2002.

[17] C. Grigor et al., "Effect of a treatment strategy of tight control for

rheumatoid arthritis (the TICORA study): A single-blind randomised controlled trial," Lancet, 2004.

[18] E. Krock, A. Jurczak, and C. I. Svensson, "Pain pathogenesis in rheumatoid arthritis-what have we learned from animal models?," Pain. 2018.

[19] D. W. Gilroy and D. Bishop-Bailey, "Lipid mediators in immune regulation and resolution," British Journal of Pharmacology. 2019.

[20] M. F. Yam, Y. C. Loh, C. S. Tan, S. K. Adam, N. A. Manan, and R. Basir, "General pathways of pain sensation and the major neurotransmitters involved in pain regulation," International Journal of Molecular Sciences. 2018.

[21] F. A. Pinho-Ribeiro, W. A. Verri, and I. M. Chiu, "Nociceptor Sensory Neuron–Immune Interactions in Pain and Inflammation," Trends in Immunology. 2017.

[22] M. Shinoda et al., "Nerve terminals extend into the temporomandibular joint of adjuvant arthritic rats," Eur. J. Pain, 2003.

[23] Y. Yamazaki, K. Ren, M. Shimada, and K. Iwata, "Modulation of paratrigeminal nociceptive neurons following temporomandibular joint inflammation in rats," Exp. Neurol., 2008.

[24] T. M. Cunha et al., "Crucial role of neutrophils in the development of mechanical inflammatory hypernociception," J. Leukoc. Biol., 2008.

[25] N. Ghasemlou, I. M. Chiu, J. P. Julien, and C. J. Woolf, "CD11b+Ly6G- myeloid cells mediate mechanical inflammatory pain hypersensitivity," Proc. Natl. Acad. Sci. U. S. A., 2015.

[26] A. Aich, L. B. Afrin, and K. Gupta, "Mast cell-mediated mechanisms of nociception," International Journal of Molecular Sciences. 2015.

[27] W. W. Li, T. Z. Guo, D. Y. Liang, Y. Sun, W. S. Kingery, and J. D. Clark, "Substance P signaling controls mast cell activation, degranulation, and nociceptive sensitization in a rat fracture model of complex regional pain syndrome," Anesthesiology, 2012.

[28] C. Gunaydin and S. S. Bilge, "Effects of nonsteroidal anti-inflammatory drugs at the molecular level," Eurasian Journal of Medicine. 2018.

[29] S. H. FERREIRA, "Prostaglandins, Aspirin-like Drugs and Analgesia," Nat. New Biol., 1972.

[30] G. R. Souza et al., "Involvement of nuclear factor kappa B in the maintenance of persistent inflammatory hypernociception," Pharmacol. Biochem. Behav., 2015.

[31] A. Nieto-Posadas et al., "Lysophosphatidic acid directly activates TRPV1 through a C-terminal binding site," Nat. Chem. Biol., 2012.

[32] H. A. Martin, A. I. Basbaum, G. C. Kwiat, E. J. Goetzl, and J. D. Levine, "Leukotriene and prostaglandin sensitization of cutaneous high-threshold C- and A-delta mechanonociceptors in the hairy skin of rat hindlimbs," Neuroscience, 1987.

[33] C. N. Serhan, "Pro-resolving lipid mediators are leads for resolution physiology," Nature. 2014.

[34] J. X. Yue et al., "Histamine Upregulates Nav1.8 Expression in Primary Afferent Neurons via H2 Receptors: Involvement in Neuropathic Pain," CNS Neurosci. Ther., 2014.

[35] C. A. Parada, C. H. Tambeli, F. Q. Cunha, and S. H. Ferreira, "The major

role of peripheral release of histamine and 5-hydroxytryptamine in formalin-induced nociception," Neuroscience, 2001.

[36] S. H. Ferreira, B. B. Lorenzetti, A. F. Bristow, and S. Poole, "Interleukin-1β as a potent hyperalgesic agent antagonized by a tripeptide analogue," Nature, 1988.

[37] A. M. Binshtok et al., "Nociceptors are interleukin-1β sensors," J. Neurosci., 2008.

[38] M. Ebbinghaus et al., "The role of interleukin-1β in arthritic pain: Main involvement in thermal, but not mechanical, hyperalgesia in rat antigen-induced arthritis," Arthritis Rheum., 2012.

[39] P. Malsch et al., "Deletion of interleukin-6 signal transducer gp130 in small sensory neurons attenuates mechanonociception and down-regulates TRPA1 expression," J. Neurosci., 2014.

[40] E. S. Fernandes et al., "A distinct role for transient receptor potential ankyrin 1, in addition to transient receptor potential vanilloid 1, in tumor necrosis factor α-induced inflammatory hyperalgesia and Freund's complete adjuvant-induced monarthritis," Arthritis Rheum., 2011.

[41] G. D. Nicol, J. C. Lopshire, and C. M. Pafford, "Tumor necrosis factor enhances the capsaicin sensitivity of rat sensory neurons," J. Neurosci., 1997.

[42] S. Gudes, O. Barkai, Y. Caspi, B. Katz, S. Lev, and A. M. Binshtok, "The role of slow and persistent ttx-resistant sodium currents in acute tumor necrosis factor-α-mediated increase in nociceptors excitability," J. Neurophysiol., 2015.

[43] F. Richter et al., "Interleukin-17 sensitizes joint nociceptors to mechanical stimuli and contributes to arthritic pain through neuronal interleukin-17 receptors in rodents," Arthritis Rheum., 2012.

[44] L. G. Pinto et al., "IL-17 mediates articular hypernociception in antigen-induced arthritis in mice," Pain, 2010.

[45] M. A. Eskander et al., "Persistent nociception triggered by nerve growth factor (NGF) is mediated by TRPV1 and oxidative mechanisms," J. Neurosci., 2015.

[46] L. S. Ro, S. T. Chen, L. M. Tang, and J. M. Jacobs, "Effect of NGF and anti-NGF on neuropathic pain in rats following chronic constriction injury of the sciatic nerve," Pain, 1999.

[47] W. H. Bos et al., "Arthritis development in patients with arthralgia is strongly associated with anti-citrullinated protein antibody status: A prospective cohort study," Ann. Rheum. Dis., 2010.

[48] G. Wigerblad et al., "Autoantibodies to citrullinated proteins induce joint pain independent of inflammation via a chemokine-dependent mechanism," Ann. Rheum. Dis., 2016.

[49] K. L. Druce, G. T. Jones, G. J. MacFarlane, and N. Basu, "Determining pathways to improvements in fatigue in rheumatoid arthritis: Results from the British Society for Rheumatology Biologics Register for rheumatoid arthritis," Arthritis Rheumatol., 2015.

[50] K. W. Drossaers-Bakker et al., "Long-term outcome in rheumatoid arthritis: A simple algorithm of baseline parameters can predict radiographic damage, disability, and disease course at 12-year followup," Arthritis Rheum., 2002.

[51] A. Judge et al., "Predictors of outcomes of total knee replacement surgery," Rheumatol. (United Kingdom), 2012.

[52] E. Nikiphorou et al., "Hand and foot surgery rates in rheumatoid arthritis have declined from 1986 to 2011, but large-joint replacement rates remain unchanged: Results from two UK inception cohorts," Arthritis Rheumatol., 2014.

[53] T. Sokka, A. Kankainen, and P. Hannonen, "Scores for functional disability in patients with rheumatoid arthritis are correlated at higher levels with pain scores than with radiographic scores," Arthritis Rheum., 2000.

[54] S. L. Murphy, A. K. Lyden, K. Phillips, D. J. Clauw, and D. A. Williams, "Association between pain, radiographic severity, and centrally-mediated symptoms in women with knee osteoarthritis," Arthritis Care Res., 2011.

[55] A. D. Beswick, V. Wylde, R. Gooberman-Hill, A. Blom, and P. Dieppe, "What proportion of patients report long-term pain after total hip or knee replacement for osteoarthritis? A systematic review of Prospective studies in unselected patients," BMJ Open. 2012.

[56] V. Wylde, A. Sayers, A. Odutola, R. Gooberman-Hill, P. Dieppe, and A. W. Blom, "Central sensitization as a determinant of patients' benefit from total hip and knee replacement," Eur. J. Pain (United Kingdom), 2017.

[57] D. A. Walsh and D. F. McWilliams, "Mechanisms, impact and management of pain in rheumatoid arthritis," Nature Reviews Rheumatology. 2014.

[58] C. J. Woolf, S. W. N. Thompson, and A. E. King, "Prolonged primary afferent induced alterations in dorsal horn neurones, an intracellular analysis in vivo and in vitro," J. Physiol. (Paris)., 1988.

[59] M. Yunus, "Editorial Review (Thematic Issue: An Update on Central Sensitivity Syndromes and the Issues of Nosology and Psychobiology)," Curr. Rheumatol. Rev., 2015.

[60] N. Sofat, V. Ejindu, and P. Kiely, "What makes osteoarthritis painful? The evidence for local and central pain processing," Rheumatology. 2011.

[61] A. I. Basbaum, D. M. Bautista, G. Scherrer, and D. Julius, "Cellular and Molecular Mechanisms of Pain," Cell. 2009.

[62] D. F. McWilliams and D. A. Walsh, "Pain mechanisms in rheumatoid arthritis," Clin. Exp. Rheumatol., 2017.

[63] A. S. Leffler, E. Kosek, T. Lerndal, B. Nordmark, and P. Hansson, "Somatosensory perception and function of diffuse noxious inhibitory controls (DNIC) in patients suffering from rheumatoid arthritis," Eur. J. Pain, 2002.

[64] L. C. Pollard, F. Ibrahim, E. H. Choy, and D. L. Scott, "Pain thresholds in rheumatoid arthritis: The effect of tender point counts and disease duration," J. Rheumatol., 2012.

[65] Y. C. Lee et al., "The relationship between disease activity, sleep, psychiatric distress and pain sensitivity in rheumatoid arthritis: A cross-sectional study," Arthritis Res. Ther., 2009.

[66] S. D. Boyden, I. N. Hossain, A. Wohlfahrt, and Y. C. Lee, "Non-inflammatory Causes of Pain in Patients with Rheumatoid Arthritis," Current Rheumatology Reports. 2016.

[67] J. Wendler et al., "Patients with rheumatoid arthritis adapt differently to repetitive painful stimuli compared to healthy controls," J. Clin. Neurosci., 2001.

[68] M. Mms. C. O. B. I. M. R. R. E. P. Yvonne C. Lee et al., "Pain Sensitization is Associated with Disease Activity

in Rheumatoid Arthritis Patients: A Cross-Sectional Study," Arthritis Care Res (Hoboken), Feb-2018. [Online]. Available: https://www.ncbi.nlm.nih.gov/pmc/articles/PMC5654691/. [Accessed: 30-Jun-2020].

[69] M. K. Sim, D. Y. Kim, J. Yoon, D. H. Park, and Y. G. Kim, "Assessment of peripheral neuropathy in patients with rheumatoid arthritis who complain of neurologic symptoms," Ann. Rehabil. Med., 2014.

[70] V. Agarwal et al., "A clinical, electrophysiological, and pathological study of neuropathy in rheumatoid arthritis," Clin. Rheumatol., 2008.

[71] S. Ahmed, T. Magan, M. Vargas, A. Harrison, and N. Sofat, "Use of the painDETECT tool in rheumatoid arthritis suggests neuropathic and sensitization components in pain reporting," J. Pain Res., 2014.

[72] W. Häuser et al., "Fibromyalgia," Nat. Rev. Dis. Prim., 2015.

[73] S. S. Zhao, S. J. Duffield, and N. J. Goodson, "The prevalence and impact of comorbid fibromyalgia in inflammatory arthritis," Best Practice and Research: Clinical Rheumatology. 2019.

[74] L. P. Queiroz, "Worldwide Epidemiology of Fibromyalgia," Curr. Pain Headache Rep., 2013.

[75] S. J. Duffield, N. Miller, S. Zhao, and N. J. Goodson, "Concomitant fibromyalgia complicating chronic inflammatory arthritis: a systematic review and meta-analysis," Rheumatology (Oxford)., 2018.

[76] F. Wolfe and K. Michaud, "Severe Rheumatoid Arthritis (RA), Worse Outcomes, Comorbid Illness, and Sociodemographic Disadvantage Characterize RA Patients with Fibromyalgia," J. Rheumatol., 2004.

[77] V. H. Morris, S. C. Cruwys, and B. L. Kidd, "Characterisation of capsaicin-induced mechanical hyperalgesia as a marker for altered nociceptive processing in patients with rheumatoid arthritis," Pain, 1997.

[78] N. G. Shenker, R. C. Haigh, P. I. Mapp, N. Harris, and D. R. Blake, "Contralateral hyperalgesia and allodynia following intradermal capsaicin injection in man," Rheumatology, 2008.

[79] K. Wartolowska, M. G. Hough, M. Jenkinson, J. Andersson, B. P. Wordsworth, and I. Tracey, "Structural changes of the brain in rheumatoid arthritis," Arthritis Rheum., 2012.

[80] P. Flodin et al., "Intrinsic brain connectivity in chronic pain: A resting-state fMRI study in patients with rheumatoid arthritis," Front. Hum. Neurosci., 2016.

[81] T. Hummel, C. Schiessl, J. Wendler, and G. Kobal, "Peripheral and central nervous changes in patients with rheumatoid arthritis in response to repetitive painful stimulation," Int. J. Psychophysiol., 2000.

[82] P. Rainville, Q. V. H. Bao, and P. Chrétien, "Pain-related emotions modulate experimental pain perception and autonomic responses," Pain, 2005.

[83] F. Matcham, L. Rayner, S. Steer, and M. Hotopf, "The prevalence of depression in rheumatoid arthritis: A systematic review and meta-analysis," Rheumatol. (United Kingdom), 2013.

[84] P. Schweinhardt, N. Kalk, K. Wartolowska, I. Chessell, P. Wordsworth, and I. Tracey, "Investigation into the neural correlates of emotional augmentation of clinical pain," Neuroimage, 2008.

[85] R. Geenen et al., "EULAR recommendations for the health

professional's approach to pain management in inflammatory arthritis and osteoarthritis," Ann. Rheum. Dis., 2018.

[86] K. Kroenke, E. E. Krebs, and M. J. Bair, "Pharmacotherapy of chronic pain: a synthesis of recommendations from systematic reviews," Gen. Hosp. Psychiatry, 2009.

[87] J. R. Kirwan, "The effect of glucocorticoids on joint destruction in rheumatoid arthritis," N. Engl. J. Med., 1995.

[88] S. M. Van Der Kooij et al., "Patient-reported outcomes in a randomized trial comparing four different treatment strategies in recent-onset rheumatoid arthritis," Arthritis Care Res., 2009.

[89] E. C. Keystone et al., "Radiographic, Clinical, and Functional Outcomes of Treatment with Adalimumab (a Human Anti-Tumor Necrosis Factor Monoclonal Antibody) in Patients with Active Rheumatoid Arthritis Receiving Concomitant Methotrexate Therapy: A Randomized, Placebo-Controlled," Arthritis Rheum., 2004.

[90] N. B. Finnerup et al., "Pharmacotherapy for neuropathic pain in adults: A systematic review and meta-analysis," Lancet Neurol., 2015.

[91] M. Kremer, E. Salvat, A. Muller, I. Yalcin, and M. Barrot, "Antidepressants and gabapentinoids in neuropathic pain: Mechanistic insights," Neuroscience. 2016.

[92] G. J. Macfarlane et al., "EULAR revised recommendations for the management of fibromyalgia," Ann. Rheum. Dis., 2017.

[93] B. L. Richards, S. L. Whittle, and R. Buchbinder, "Neuromodulators for pain management in rheumatoid arthritis," Cochrane Database Syst. Rev., 2012.

[94] N. Sofat et al., "The effect of pregabalin or duloxetine on arthritis pain: A clinical and mechanistic study in people with hand osteoarthritis," J. Pain Res., 2017.

[95] A. C. d. C. Williams, C. Eccleston, and S. Morley, "Psychological therapies for the management of chronic pain (excluding headache) in adults," Cochrane Database of Systematic Reviews. 2012.

[96] J. A. Astin, W. Beckner, K. Soeken, M. C. Hochberg, and B. Berman, "Psychological interventions for rheumatoid arthritis: A meta-analysis of randomized controlled trials," Arthritis Rheum., 2002.

[97] K. Knittle, S. Maes, and V. De Gucht, "Psychological interventions for rheumatoid arthritis: Examining the role of self-regulation with a systematic review and meta-analysis of randomized controlled trials," Arthritis Care Res., 2010.

[98] S. Hewlett et al., "Reducing arthritis fatigue impact: Two-year randomised controlled trial of cognitive behavioural approaches by rheumatology teams (RAFT)," Ann. Rheum. Dis., 2019.

[99] L. Sharpe, "Psychosocial management of chronic pain in patients with rheumatoid arthritis: Challenges and solutions," Journal of Pain Research. 2016.

[100] A. Baillet, M. Vaillant, M. Guinot, R. Juvin, and P. Gaudin, "Efficacy of resistance exercises in rheumatoid arthritis: Meta-analysis of randomized controlled trials," Rheumatology, 2012.

Section 3

Clinical Challenges in Rheumatoid Arthritis Patients

Chapter 4

Vascular Involvement in Rheumatoid Arthritis

Alexandru Caraba, Stela Iurciuc and Mircea Iurciuc

Abstract

Rheumatoid arthritis (RA) represents the one of the most common inflammatory rheumatic diseases, which generates disability and significantly reduces the quality of life. RA can affect the vascular system, in addition to joint involvement. Vascular involvement increases the morbidity and mortality among these patients. Macrovascular disease, related to accelerated atherosclerosis, has a high prevalence among RA patients, in the form of carotid artery disease, ischemic heart disease, and peripheral arterial obstructive disease. Microvascular disease, studied in recent years by means of nailfold capillaroscopy, is present even in the early stage of RA evolution. Rheumatoid vasculitis can occur in severe forms of RA.

Keywords: macrovascular, microvascular involvement, rheumatoid arthritis

1. Introduction

Rheumatoid arthritis (RA) is a chronic inflammatory disorder, characterized by synovitis of small- and medium-sized joints, which causes cartilage breakdown, bone erosions, and finally destruction and loss of joints function. But beside the joints involvement, RA, especially with long-term evolution and suboptimal control of the disease activity, can generate systemic involvement (cardiovascular, respiratory, haematologic) [1].

RA is the most common inflammatory rheumatic disease, affecting about 0.5–1% of North American and European people over 18 years. The RA incidence and prevalence have regional differences: the lowest rates are identified in Southern regions, and the highest rates are present in Northern Europe and North America. Women are more frequently affected than men (women/men ratio 3/1), this disease occurring more commonly in the 4th or the 5th decades of life [2, 3].

RA is an autoimmune disorder; through the interaction between genetic predisposition and environmental factors, a trigger event generates an inflammatory autoimmune response, which affects primarily the synovial joint but also the blood vessels [1].

The interrelation between RA and vascular involvement began to be studied many years ago. In 2008, in their review, Szekanecz and Koch introduced the term "vascular rheumatology," referring to vascular impairment from inflammatory rheumatic diseases [4]. Indeed, in RA, vascular involvement comprises both macro- and microvessels. Special attention requires rheumatoid vasculitis, a rare but severe complication of this disease. Histologically, vascular lesions have been found in 25% of RA patients [5]. Patients with RA are prone to early and accelerated atherosclerosis, which induces higher cardiovascular risk, independent of traditional risk factors (diabetes mellitus, arterial hypertension, smoking, dyslipidemia, age, lifestyle). RA-related risk factors are identified and characterized in these patients [6, 7]. In RA patients, the cardiovascular risk is obtained by the multiplication of measured risk (SCORE, Framingham) by a factor of 1.5, if two of the three following criteria are fulfilled (RA evolution >10 years, positivity of RF or ACPA, extra-articular involvement) [8].

2. Risk factors for vascular involvement

Vascular involvement in RA patients has a multifactorial model. Traditional cardiovascular risk factors together with those related to RA contribute to the development of macro- and microvascular involvement. It is known that the first step in atherogenesis development is endothelial dysfunction. Several factors associated with RA are involved in the endothelial dysfunction appearance: pro-inflammatory mediators and cells, oxidative stress, insulin resistance, physical inactivity, genetic factors, and drugs [9].

During its evolution, RA is a chronic inflammatory condition. Even in the preclinical stage, then continuing with the period when the clinical picture is complete, the chronic inflammatory environment exists in these patients. Pro-inflammatory cytokines contribute to synovial inflammation and to atherosclerosis development, through endothelial dysfunction.

Under physiological conditions, endothelium represents an active barrier between vascular wall and bloodstream, being involved in maintaining vascular muscle tone and homeostasis, controlling cell adhesion, proliferation, and coagulation balance. In pathophysiological conditions (chronic inflammatory diseases), these endothelium physiological functions are disturbed, and endothelial dysfunction occurs. During this new situation, reduced vasodilation, pro-inflammatory and prothrombotic status, and increased cell adhesion and proliferation contribute to atherosclerosis development. Endothelial dysfunction is a preclinical marker of atherosclerosis development, commonly detected in RA patients, but it is also involved in plaque progression and the occurrence of atherosclerotic complications [10, 11]. In RA patients, endothelial dysfunction occurs differentially in different vascular beds (macro- and microcirculation) [12]. Bocci et al. showed that in RA patients, the coronary microvascular involvement is identified in the absence of macrovascular disease [13].

Several factors are involved in endothelial dysfunction appearance in RA patients (**Table 1**) [9, 11].

2.1 Arterial hypertension

High blood pressure represents an independent predictor of cardiovascular events in RA patients. COMORA study reported that the prevalence of high blood pressure among RA patients was about 40% [14]. In their meta-analysis, Baghdadi et al. reported that high blood pressure was associated with a relative risk of cardiovascular morbidity of 2.24 in patients with RA [15]. On the other hand, Panoulas et al. identified that the most important determinant of target organ damage in RA patients is arterial hypertension [16]. It is known that the increase in systolic blood pressure with 20 mmHg is associated with high risk of endothelial dysfunction and cardiovascular disease. Some drugs used in RA therapy, as Leflunomide, NSAIDs, corticoids, and cyclosporine, are associated with high risk of arterial hypertension development, with consecutive endothelial dysfunction [7]. In hypertensive RA patients, ambulatory blood pressure monitoring revealed that the non-dipper and excessive dipper

Traditional risk factors
• Arterial hypertension
• Dyslipidemia
• Insulin resistance and metabolic syndrome
• Obesity
• Smoking
RA-related factors
• Chronic inflammatory status
• Oxidative stress

Table 1.
Factors involved in RA endothelial dysfunction.

patterns were frequent among them and pulse pressure was increased, these characteristics predisposing to cardiovascular complications [17]. Most researchers wondered if high blood pressure is effectively controlled in RA patients. Panoulas et al. and Desai et al., in their studies, showed that the identification and effective control of high blood pressure is suboptimal in RA patients [18, 19]. Two studies published in 2016 and one published in 2019 showed that there were no significant differences in the diagnosis and therapy of high blood pressure in RA patients versus the general population [20–22].

2.2 Dyslipidemia

Dyslipidemia represents a well-known traditional cardiovascular risk factor, affecting between 55 and 65% of the RA patients [23]. These patients present low levels of low density lipoprotein (LDL), high density lipoprotein (HDL), and total cholesterol, these levels being inversely correlated with markers of inflammation. But during inflammation, these molecules develop functional and structural changes, becoming atherogenic and promoting endothelial dysfunction. Some drugs used in RA treatment may increase lipid levels: DMARDs, TNF-α inhibitors, tocilizumab, and IL-6 receptor blocker [8].

2.3 Insulin resistance and metabolic syndrome

The prevalence of insulin resistance and metabolic syndrome is increased in RA patients (40%), increasing the risk of endothelial dysfunction and cardiovascular events by twofold compared to the general population. RA with high activity increases the effect of insulin resistance/metabolic syndrome on endothelial dysfunction. The effect of the medication that decreases the RA activity (DMARDs, biologics) on insulin resistance is not to be neglected. Endothelial-dependent vasodilation, mediated by nitric oxide release, is impaired in insulin resistance individuals. They display high levels of endothelin and plasminogen activator inhibitor in plasma [8].

2.4 Obesity

Obesity, physical inactivity, and endothelial dysfunction coexist in RA patients. Obesity is associated with other cardiovascular risk factors, as atherogenic dyslipidemia, high blood pressure, insulin resistance, and low grade inflammation, generating endothelial dysfunction. But in RA an association between low body mass (secondary to high rheumatoid inflammation, generating rheumatoid cachexia) and cardiovascular events, too, is described [8].

2.5 Smoking

Another cardiovascular risk factor, smoking, is involved in RA appearance [24]. Rojas-Serrano et al. showed that the RA patients who smoked had a more severe RA evolution and positivity for rheumatoid factor and anticitrullinated protein antibodies [25]. Baghdadi et al. demonstrated that the cardiovascular risk was higher in RA patients who smoked [15].

Baghdadi et al. revealed in their meta-analysis that in RA patients the increased cardiovascular morbidity is related to the presence of high blood pressure [relative risk (RR): 2.24, 95% confidence intervals (CI): 1.42–3.06], smoking (RR: 1.5, 95% CI: 1.15–1.84), obesity (RR: 1.16, 95% CI: 1.03–1.29), insulin resistance (RR: 1.94, 95% CI: 1.58–2.30), and atherogenic dyslipidemia (RR: 1.73, 95% CI: 1.03–2.44) [15].

2.6 Inflammation

Chronic inflammation is considered to be an independent risk factor for the atherosclerosis development. Together with immune dysregulation, it contributes to endothelial dysfunction and atheroma plaque development. The cardiovascular risk begins to be evident from the early stages of RA, making the cardiovascular investigation necessary even from the first medical visit [26].

Chronic inflammation is considered to be of utmost importance in endothelial dysfunction onset. The previous studies have shown that the inflammatory processes in the rheumatoid synovium and atherosclerotic plaques are remarkably similar. TNF-alpha, interleukin-1 (IL-1), and interleukin-6 (IL-6) play an important role in RA pathogenesis, but they are involved in the development of endothelial dysfunction, too. TNF-alpha increases IL-1, IL-6, IL-8, and chemokines synthesis. On the other hand, this cytokine increases cellular infiltration in the synovium, through enhancing chemokine expression, endothelial cells activation, and neoangiogenesis. IL-1 stimulates the expression of adhesion molecules on the endothelial cells and neoangiogenesis. IL-6 contributes to endothelial cell activation; upregulates the expression of the chemokines that attract T cells, leading to enhanced cellular infiltration; and increases the concentration of VEGF with high vascular permeability appearance. VEGF induces the endothelial cell activation and differentiation, generating neoangiogenesis, too. These cytokines have metabolic effects, acting on the adipose tissue, the skeletal muscle, and the liver and contributing to the traditional cardiovascular risk factor production (insulin resistance, obesity). They contribute to the endothelial dysfunction development.

The inflammatory environment increases the effect of traditional cardiovascular risk factors on endothelial cells, generating endothelial dysfunction development. Other studies revealed that the anti-inflammatory treatment improves the endothelial dysfunction in RA patients [8, 27, 28].

2.7 Reactive oxygen species

Reactive oxygen species (ROS), generated at higher concentrations at sites of inflammation, can induce cellular injury. Vascular endothelial cells represent the main target for the ROS, increasing the endothelial permeability and promoting leukocyte adhesion. On the other hand, high levels of ROS and low levels of antioxidants in RA with high inflammatory activity generate the impairment of the HDL function. Through these effects, ROS contributes to the endothelial dysfunction appearance in RA patients [7, 10].

2.8 RA treatment and vascular dysfunction

The drugs used in RA therapy may contribute to vascular dysfunction and cardiovascular risk.

Nonsteroidal anti-inflammatory drugs (NSAIDs) represent a class of drugs frequently used by these patients. The data regarding the NSAID use and cardiovascular risk in RA patients remain controversial. Data from the Danish nationwide registry revealed that the increased cardiovascular risk related to the overall use of NSAIDs in RA patients was modest and even significantly lower than in non-RA subjects. Rofecoxib and diclofenac were the exception, being associated with increased cardiovascular risk [29]. It is recommended to use NSAIDs with caution in RA patients in the presence of cardiovascular risk factors or in the presence of ischemic cardiovascular disease [8, 9].

Corticosteroids contribute to insulin resistance, high blood pressure, and atherogenic dyslipidemia; all these factors are associated with endothelial dysfunction and subsequently appearance of cardiovascular events. But, on the other hand, by controlling inflammation, corticoids may reduce cardiovascular risk in RA patients. EULAR recommended the corticoid use at lowest dose possible (<7.5 mg Prednisone/day), for the shortest period of time [9].

Among disease-modifying drugs (DMARDs), methotrexate, sulfasalazine, and hydroxychloroquine are associated with the cardiovascular risk reduction. By controlling inflammation (decrease of pro-inflammatory cytokine level), methotrexate improves the endothelial function in RA patients. But this drug contributes to endothelial protection by means of induction of AMPK-regulated protective genes. Sulfasalazine interferes with platelet function. Hydroxychloroquine improves lipid profile and has antithrombotic effects, thus reducing the cardiovascular risk. Leflunomide and cyclosporine are associated with arterial hypertension.

By using biologics (anti-TNF-alpha, anti-CD28, anti-CD20, anti-IL 6, anti-IL1), cardiovascular risk was reduced comparatively with the RA patients without this therapy.

Anti-TNF-alpha therapy improves endothelial function by means of inflammation reduction. It is important to know that the reduction in cardiovascular risk was recorded only in patients responsive to anti-TNF-alpha treatment.

Anti-IL-6 therapy improves endothelial function (measured by means of flow-mediated vasodilation) very early during the treatment. This effect is determined by reducing inflammation, although total cholesterol, LDL-cholesterol, and triglyceride levels are increased.

Anti-CD20 therapy reduces RA activity and has favorable effects on lipid profile, reducing endothelial dysfunction.

The use of abatacept in RA treatment has generated conflicting data regarding vascular dysfunction. Tofacitinib increases total cholesterol levels but without change of atherogenic index. This new drug was associated with low rates of cardiovascular events in RA patients [1, 8].

3. Macro- and microvascular endothelial dysfunction

All these factors contribute to disruption of vascular environment at the macro- and microcirculation levels, occurring endothelial dysfunction [2, 7].

Morphological assessment	
Conducting artery	Carotid intima-media thickness (cIMT)
Capillaries	Nailfold capillaroscopy
Functional assessment	
Conduit artery	Pulse wave velocity (PWV) Pulse wave analysis (PWA) Flow-mediated dilation (FMD) Nitroglycerin-mediated dilation (NMD)
Arterioles	Laser Doppler imaging with iontophoresis Venous occlusion plethysmography

Table 2.
Methods for morphologic and functional vascular assessment.

Macrovascular and microvascular endothelial dysfunction is identified in RA patients, not associated with each other, increasing cardiovascular risk in these patients [30]. The studies revealed a weak correlation between microvascular and macrovascular endothelial dysfunction in RA patients. Microvascular endothelial dysfunction results from the interaction between inflammation, immune dysregulation, and traditional cardiovascular risk factors, representing a significant factor related to accelerated atherosclerosis and future cardiovascular events in RA patients [31].

Structural and functional assessment of vasculature in RA patients uses different methods (**Table 2**). It is known that the functional and morphological vascular changes may coexist, especially in the early atherosclerosis [27].

4. Macrovascular involvement in RA

Endothelial dysfunction is present in RA patients compared to healthy controls. Although not all studies have shown the connection between endothelial dysfunction and inflammation, the use of specific RA medication (especially anti-TNF-alpha) has improved endothelial function in RA patients [32].

Arterial stiffness is increased in RA patients compared with controls, but an association between arterial stiffness and disease activity was not highlighted [27, 32].

Most studies identified that the cIMT was increased in RA patients, even in cases with newly established diagnosis. cIMT increases with the disease duration but is well known that the increase of cIMT is associated with the age of patients. The most studies did not reveal a consistent link between inflammation and vascular parameters. Van Zanten et al. explained that the long-standing, not current inflammation has had vascular impact in RA patients [33]. Carotid plaque (**Figure 1**) is common findings among RA patients. Roman et al. reported that the carotid plaque was three times more prevalent in RA patients than in controls [34]. Dessein et al. identified that the 31% of RA patients had carotid plaque [35]. Another study, performed by Pope et al., reported a prevalence of carotid atherosclerotic plaque about 35% in RA patients [36]. Protogerou et al. highlighted the importance of carotid ultrasonography associated with the femoral one in RA cardiovascular risk assessment [37].

Plaque rupture leads to the occurrence of clinical events. The risk of plaque rupture is determined by its composition (calcification, lipid-rich necrotic core, neovascularization, inflammatory cell infiltration) and, on the other hand, by the

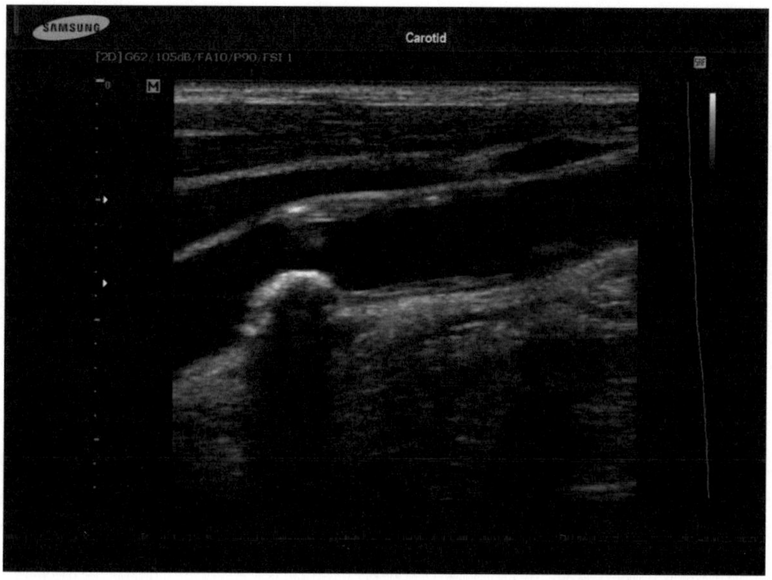

Figure 1.
Common carotid artery: Ultrasonography (increased cIMT and plaques in a long-standing RA evolution; personal collection).

presence of inflammation. Pro-inflammatory cytokines (IL-6, TNF-alpha) are related to plaque progression and the appearance of complications [32, 35]. Skeoch et al. demonstrated in their study the increased prevalence of atherosclerosis in RA, providing data to confirm that atheroma plaques are at high risk of complications [38].

Ruscitti et al. have shown increased incidence and prevalence of subclinical and clinical atherosclerosis in RA patients, but reaching and maintaining remission had positive effect on the atherogenesis development [39].

Further longitudinal studies are necessary in order to characterize the accelerated atherosclerosis in RA patients [32].

5. Microvascular involvement in RA

Yki-Jarvinen et al. studied the microvascular endothelial function in RA patients, using intrabrachial artery infusions of acetylcholine (endothelium dependent vasodilation) and sodium nitroprusside (endothelium independent vasodilation). The authors concluded that the basal blood flow was increased, correlated with the degree of RA inflammatory activity and more inhibited by NG-monomethyl-L-arginine, suggesting that the responsiveness to nitric oxide was reduced [40]. In another study, Galarraga et al. identified that the systemic inflammation (evaluated by serum levels of C-reactive protein) was independently associated with microvascular dysfunction in RA patients [41]. Studying 65 RA patients and 40 healthy controls, Arosio et al. showed that the RA patients presented impaired microcirculatory reactivity, endothelial dysfunction, and increased arterial stiffness. The authors concluded that these vascular alterations would be the link between RA and cardiovascular morbidity and mortality [42]. Endothelial dysfunction in RA patients was associated with high values of C-reactive protein and inducible nitric oxide synthase [43].

Microvascular morphological assessment may be performed by nailfold capillaroscopy, a noninvasive and repeatable method. By using this method, the following parameters are evaluated: tortuosity, loop size, density, angiogenesis, capillary loss, microbleeding, subpapillary venous plexus, and architectural structure [44].

McGill and Gow studied by nailfold capillaroscopy the microvascular changes in patients with systemic sclerosis (10 pts.), systemic lupus erythematosus (9 pts.), and rheumatoid arthritis (11 pts.). They reported that the nailfold capillaroscopy had a specificity of 89% and a sensitivity of 80% in the differentiation of the capillaroscopic models of these three diseases [45]. In another study, performed by Altomonte et al., the authors identified that in RA patients the common capillaroscopic changes were represented by elongation and capillary tortuosity. Besides them, the visibility of the subpapillary venous plexus was correlated with the endothelial dysfunction [46]. In the study performed on 80 RA patients and 30 healthy controls, Kuryliszyn-Moskal identified a significant correlation between soluble CD4 levels and the capillaroscopy findings [47].

In present, it is considered that there is no specific capillaroscopic model for RA [48]. Elongated and tiny loops, microhemorrhages, capillary low density, and subpapillary venous plexus visibility are common among RA patients [5].

Microvascular involvement appears early in the RA evolution. In their study, Scardina and Messina revealed that in patients with early RA, labial mucosa capillaries presented alterations, as: elongation, decreased capillaries caliber compared to healthy subjects. The authors suggested that the microvascular alterations could be extremely important in the diagnosis of suspected RA patients [5].

In their article, Lin et al. presented that in RA, the most common findings were represented by elongated and tiny capillaries and capillary tortuosity. The subpapillary venous plexus was visualized in RA patients who had antinuclear antibodies [44]. Sag et al. analyzed nailfold findings in 201 RA patients and 50 healthy controls. The authors examined the relationship between nailfold capillaroscopic findings and disease activity, expressed as DAS28. In 45.77% of RA patients, the authors identified nonspecific capillaroscopy findings: tortuosity, dilated capillaries, and bushy capillaries. The association of Raynaud's phenomenon increased the incidence of nailfold capillaroscopy abnormalities. No relation was found between microvascular abnormalities and RA activity score [49] (**Figure 2**).

Bernardino et al. identified mainly a non-scleroderma capillaroscopic pattern in RA patients. The authors suggested that the microvascular abnormalities identified in RA patients represented the results of inflammation and endothelial dysfunction [50]. Cutolo et al. highlighted that in RA patients "scleroderma-like" capillaroscopic pattern may be found, especially in association with rheumatoid vasculitis [51].

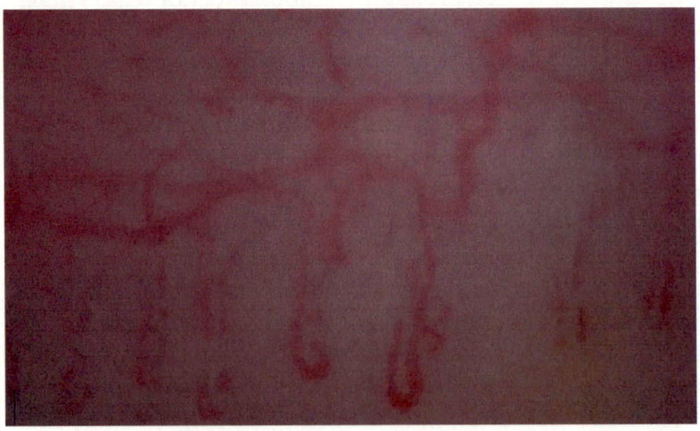

Figure 2.
Nailfold capillaroscopy (×200; subpapillary venous plexus visible, fragmentation of capillary blood circulation in patient with early RA; personal collection).

6. Rheumatoid vasculitis

Rheumatoid vasculitis (RV) is the most serious extra-articular complication of RA with long-term evolution, generating high rates of morbidity and mortality (up to 40%, during 5 years) [52].

It can affect any organ or system, but the most frequent involved are the skin (nailfold lesions, palpable purpura, and leg ulcers) and peripheral nervous system (mononeuritis multiplex, distal symmetric sensory or sensorimotor neuropathy) [53–55].

Due to earlier diagnosis and new therapeutic strategies for RA, the prevalence of RV had progressively reduced over time. RV appears in RA patients with severe immunological abnormalities, associating with other extra-articular manifestations [1].

RV is characterized by inflammation of small- and medium-sized arteries and capillaries. The risk factors associated with RV are represented by RA with prolonged evolution (> 10 years), rheumatoid nodules, males, smoking, seropositivity of rheumatoid factor, HLA-DRB1*0401/*0401, *0401/*0404, and *0101/*0401, HLA-C3 [55, 56].

RV can affect any organ or system of the body [1].

Clinical features of RV are cutaneous manifestations (digital infarcts, livedo reticularis, palpable purpura, ulcers, painful nodules, or even digital gangrene), peripheral nervous system manifestations (mononeuritis multiplex, distal symmetric sensory or sensorimotor neuropathy), and internal organ manifestations (due to coronary, cerebral, mesenteric, renal artery involvement, much less common, but with significant morbidity and mortality). The patients with Felty's syndrome develop more frequent RV [1, 54, 56].

Laboratory features of RV are represented by high levels of sedimentation rate and C-reactive protein, thrombocytosis, anemia, high levels of anti-cyclic citrullinated peptide antibodies and rheumatoid factor, and decreased levels of complement in patients with RV than the patients without this complication [1, 56, 57].

The RV diagnosis is easily established in the presence of cutaneous or nervous manifestations. Internal organ manifestations represent a challenge in establishing the correct RV diagnosis. Diagnosis confirmation is established by histopathological examination of the involved skin, muscle, nerve, or another affected organ [56].

In present, there are no guidelines for the RV treatment. Corticosteroids and cyclophosphamide have been used in severe, life-threatening cases of RV. In milder forms of RV, corticosteroids and methotrexate or azathioprine have been used. Rituximab and corticosteroids are preferred, due to higher efficiency and lower toxicity [55, 58, 59].

7. Conclusion

Vascular involvement in RA patients remains a chapter open to further research, in order to develop preventive measures, early diagnosis, and efficient therapy.

Conflict of interest

The authors declare no conflict of interest.

Author details

Alexandru Caraba[1*], Stela Iurciuc[2] and Mircea Iurciuc[2]

1 Division of Rheumatology, Department of Internal Medicine, University of Medicine and Pharmacy "Victor Babeş", Timişoara, Romania

2 Department of Cardiology, University of Medicine and Pharmacy "Victor Babeş", Timişoara, Romania

*Address all correspondence to: alexcaraba@yahoo.com

References

[1] Padjen I, Gabay C, Aletaha D. Pathogenesis and clinical aspects of rheumatoid arthritis. In: Bijlsma JWJ, Hachula E, editors. Textbook on Rheumatic Disease. 3rd ed. London: BMJ Publishing Group Ltd; 2018. pp. 237-275

[2] Rajaei A, Dehghan P, Amiri A. Nail fold capillaroscopy in 430 patients with rheumatoid arthritis. Caspian Journal of Internal Medicine. 2017;**8**(4):269-275

[3] Safiri S, Kolahi AA, Hoy D, Smith E, Bettampadi D, et al. Global, regional and national burden of rheumatoid arthritis 1990-2017: A systematic analysis of the global burden of disease study 2017. Annals of the Rheumatic Diseases. 2019;**78**:1463-1471

[4] Szekanecz Z, Koch AE. Vascular involvement in rheumatic diseases: 'vascular rheumatology'. Arthritis Research & Therapy. 2008;**10**:224. DOI: 10.1186/ar2515

[5] Scardina GA, Messina P. Microvascular abnormalities in patients with rheumatoid arthritis. Annals of Anatomy. 2006;**188**(5):425-429. DOI: 10.1016/j.aanat.2006.04.004

[6] Das S, Padhan P. An overview of the extraarticular involvement in rheumatoid arthritis and its management. Journal of Pharmacology and Pharmacotherapeutics. 2017;**8**:81-86

[7] Rawla P. Cardiac and vascular complications in rheumatoid arthritis. Reumatologia. 2019;**57**(1):27-36. DOI: 10.5114/reum.2019.83236

[8] Zegkos T, Kitas G, Dimitroulas T. Cardiovascular risk in rheumatoid arthritis: Assessment, management and next steps. Therapeutic Advances in Musculoskeletal Disease. 2016;**8**(3):86-101

[9] Agca R, Heslinga SC, Rollefstad S, Heslinga M, McInnes IB, et al. EULAR recommendations for cardiovascular disease risk management in patients with rheumatoid arthritis and other forms of inflammatory joint disorders: 2015/2016 update. Annals of the Rheumatic Diseases. 2017;**76**:17-28

[10] Hadi HAR, Carr CS, Suwaidi JA. Endothelial dysfunction: Cardiovascular risk factors, therapy, and outcome. Vascular Health and Risk Management. 2005;**1**(3):183-198

[11] Versari D, Daghini E, Virdis A, Ghiadoni L, Taddei S. Endothelial dysfunction as a target for prevention of cardiovascular disease. Diabetes Care. 2009;**32**(Suppl 2):S314-S321

[12] Hill CE, Phillips JK, Sandow SL. Heterogeneous control of blood flow amongst different vascular beds. Medicinal Research Reviews. 2001;**21**(1):1-60

[13] Bocci EB, Delle Monache F, Cesarotti M, Angrisani C, Gerli R. Recent views on the pathogenesis of cardiovascular damage associated with rheumatoid arthritis. Recenti Progressi in Medicina. 2005;**96**(2):65-120

[14] Dougados M, Soubrier M, Antunez A, Balint P, Balsa A, et al. Prevalence of comorbidities in rheumatoid arthritis and evaluation of their monitoring: Results of an international, crosssectional study (COMORA). Annals of the Rheumatic Diseases. 2014;**73**:62-68

[15] Baghdadi L, Woodman R, Shanahan E, Mangoni A. The impact of traditional cardiovascular risk factors on cardiovascular outcomes in patients with rheumatoid arthritis: A systematic review and meta-analysis. PLoS One. 2015;**10**:e0117952

[16] Panoulas VF, Toms TE, Metsios GS, Stavropoulos-Kalinoglou A, Kosovitsas A, et al. Target organ damage in patients with rheumatoid arthritis: The role of blood pressure and heart rate. Atherosclerosis. 2010;**209**:255-260

[17] Rihacek I, Nemec P, Rihacek M, Kianicka B, Berukstis A, et al. Ambulatory blood pressure monitoring and hypertension related cardiovascular risk in patients with rheumatoid arthritis. International Journal of Clinical Rheumatology. 2017;**12**(6):142-150

[18] Panoulas VF, Douglas KM, Milionis HJ, Stavropoulos-Kalinglou A, Nightingale P, et al. Prevalence and associations of hypertension and its control in patients with rheumatoid arthritis. Rheumatology. 2007;**46**:1477-1482

[19] Desai SS, Myles JD, Kaplan MJ. Suboptimal cardiovascular risk factor identification and management in patients with rheumatoid arthritis: A cohort analysis. Arthritis Research & Therapy. 2012;**14**:R270

[20] Alemao E, Cawston H, Bourhis F, Al M, Rutten-van Mölken MP, et al. Cardiovascular risk factor management in patients with RA compared to matched non-RA patients. Rheumatology. 2016;**55**:809-816

[21] An J, Cheetham TC, Reynolds K, Alemao E, Kawabata H, et al. Traditional cardiovascular disease risk factor management in rheumatoid arthritis compared to matched nonrheumatoid arthritis in a US managed care setting. Arthritis Care and Research. 2016;**68**:629-637

[22] Boersma P, McElwee MK, Hashmi H, Schreiner P, Demmer RT, Shmagel A. Blood pressure trends in patients with seropositive rheumatoid arthritis compared with controls without rheumatoid arthritis: A retrospective cohort study. ACR Open Rheumatology. 2019;**1**(3):173-181. DOI: 10.1002/acr2.1029

[23] Toms T, Symmons D, Kitas G. Dyslipidaemia in rheumatoid arthritis: The role of inflammation, drugs, lifestyle and genetic factors. Current Vascular Pharmacology. 2010; **8**:301-326

[24] Bergstrom U, Jacobsson L, Nilsson J, Berglund G, Turesson C. Pulmonary dysfunction, smoking, socioeconomic status and the risk of developing rheumatoid arthritis. Rheumatology. 2011;**50**:2005-2013

[25] Rojas-Serrano J, Perez L, Garcia C, Moctezuma F, Álvarez-Hernández E, et al. Current smoking status is associated to a non-ACR 50 response in early rheumatoid arthritis. A cohort study. Clinical Rheumatology. 2011;**30**:1589-1593

[26] Aziz M, Yadav KS. Atherosclerosis: An extraarticular manifestation of rheumatoid arthritis. Annals of Clinical and Laboratory Research. 2016;**4**:4

[27] Sandoo A, van Zanten JJCSV, Metsios GS, Carroll D, Kitas GD. Vascular function and morphology in rheumatoid arthritis: A systematic review. Rheumatology. 2011;**50**: 2125-2139. DOI: 10.1093/rheumatology/ker275

[28] Yang XZ, Chang Y, Wei W. Endothelial dysfunction and inflammation: Immunity in rheumatoid arthritis. Mediators of Inflammation. 2016;**2016**:6813016. DOI: 10.1155/2016/6813016

[29] Lindhardsen J, Gislason G, Jacobsen S, Ahlehoff O, Olsen A, et al. Non-steroidal antiinflammatory drugs and risk of cardiovascular disease in patients with rheumatoid arthritis: A nationwide cohort study. Annals of the Rheumatic Diseases. 2013;**73**:1515-1521

[30] Sandoo A, Carroll D, Metsios GS, Kitas GD, van Zanten VJJ. The association between microvascular and macrovascular endothelial function in patients with rheumatoid arthritis: A cross-sectional study. Arthritis Research & Therapy. 2011;**13**:R99

[31] Erre GL, Piga M, Fedele AL, Mura S, Piras A, et al. Prevalence and determinants of peripheral microvascular endothelial dysfunction in rheumatoid arthritis patients: A multicenter cross-sectional study. Mediators of Inflammation. 2018;**2018**:6548715. DOI: 10.1155/2018/6548715

[32] Dimitroulas T, Sandoo A, Skeoch S, O'Sullivan M, Yessirkepov M, et al. Rheumatoid arthritis. In: Nussinovitch U, editor. The Heart in Rheumatic, Autoimmune and Inflammatory Diseases. Elsevier; 2017. pp. 129-165

[33] van Zanten VJJ, Kitas GD. Inflammation, carotid intima-media thickness and atherosclerosis in rheumatoid arthritis. Arthritis Research & Therapy. 2008;**10**:102

[34] Roman MJ, Moeller E, Davis A, Paget SA, Crow MK, et al. Preclinical carotid atherosclerosis in patients with rheumatoid arthritis. Annals of Internal Medicine. 2006;**144**(4):249-256. DOI: 10.7326/0003-4819-144-4-200602210-00006

[35] Dessein PH, Joffe BI, Veller MG, Stevens BA, Tobias M, et al. Traditional and nontraditional cardiovascular risk factors are associated with atherosclerosis in rheumatoid arthritis. The Journal of Rheumatology. 2005;**32**(3):435-442

[36] Pope JE, Nevskaya T, Barra L, Parraga G. Carotid artery atherosclerosis in patients with active rheumatoid arthritis: Predictors of plaque occurrence and progression over 24 weeks. The Open Rheumatology Journal. 2016;**10**:49-59. DOI: 10.2174/1874312901610010049

[37] Protogerou AD, Fransen J, Zampeli E, Argyris AA, Aissopou E, et al. The additive value of femoral ultrasound for subclinical atherosclerosis assessment in a single center cohort of 962 adults, including high risk patients with rheumatoid arthritis, human immunodeficiency virus infection and type 2 diabetes mellitus. PLoS One. 2015;**10**(7):e0132307. DOI: 10.1371/journal.pone.0132307

[38] Skeoch S, Cristinacce PLH, Williams H, Pemberton P, Xu D, et al. Imaging atherosclerosis in rheumatoid arthritis: Evidence for increased prevalence, altered phenotype and a link between systemic and localised plaque inflammation. Scientific Reports. 2017;**7**(1):827. DOI: 10.1038/s41598-017-00989-w

[39] Ruscitti P, Cipriani P, Liakouli V, Iacono D, Pantano I, et al. Subclinical and clinical atherosclerosis in rheumatoid arthritis: Results from the 3-year, multicentre, prospective, observational GIRRCS (*Gruppo Italiano di Ricerca in Reumatologia Clinica e Sperimentale*) study. Arthritis Research & Therapy. 2019;**21**:204. DOI: 10.1186/s13075-019-1975-y

[40] Yki-Jarvinen H, Bergholm R, Leirisalo-Repo M. Increased inflammatory activity parallels increased basal nitric oxide production and blunted response to nitric oxide in vivo in rheumatoid arthritis. Annals of the Rheumatic Diseases. 2003;**62**:630-634

[41] Galarraga B, Khan F, Kumar P, Pullar T, Belch JJ. C-reactive protein: The underlying cause of microvascular dysfunction in rheumatoid arthritis. Rheumatology. 2008;**47**:1780-1784

[42] Arosio E, De Marchi S, Rigoni A, Prior M, Delva P, Lechi A. Forearm

haemodynamics, arterial stiffness and microcirculatory reactivity in rheumatoid arthritis. Journal of Hypertension. 2007;**25**:1273-1278

[43] Maki-Petaja KM, Cheriyan J, Booth AD, Hall FC, Brown J, et al. Inducible nitric oxide synthase activity is increased in patients with rheumatoid arthritis and contributes to endothelial dysfunction. International Journal of Cardiology. 2008;**129**:399-405

[44] Lin KM, Cheng TT, Chen CJ. Clinical applications of nailfold capillaroscopy in different rheumatic diseases. Journal of Internal Medicine of Taiwan. 2009;**20**:238-247

[45] McGill NW, Gow PJ. Nailfold capillaroscopy: A blinded study of its discriminatory value in scleroderma, systemic lupus erythematosus, and rheumatoid arthritis. Australian and New Zealand Journal of Medicine. 1986;**16**(4):457-460. DOI: 10.1111/j.1445-5994.1986.tb02010.x

[46] Altomonte L, Zoli A, Galossi A, Mirone L, Tulli A, et al. Microvascular capillaroscopic abnormalities in rheumatoid arthritis patients. Clinical and Experimental Rheumatology. 1995;**13**:83-86

[47] Kuryliszyn-Moskal A. Cytokines and soluble CD4 and CD8 molecules in rheumatoid arthritis: Relationship to systematic vasculitis and microvascular capillaroscopic abnormalities. Clinical Rheumatology. 1998;**17**(6):489

[48] Ali AM, Hamza SM, Aboud FM, El-Shahat NM. Nailfold capillaroscopic changes in Egyptian patients with psoriatic arthritis in comparison to rheumatoid arthritis. The Egyptian Rheumatologist. 2019;**41**:303-307

[49] Sag S, Sag MS, Tekeoglu I, Kamanli A, Nas K, Aydın Y. Nailfold videocapillaroscopy results in patients with rheumatoid arthritis. Clinical Rheumatology. 2017;**36**(9):1969-1974. DOI: 10.1007/s10067-017-3696-4

[50] Bernardino V, Rodrigues A, Lladó A, Panarra A. Nailfold capillaroscopy and autoimmune connective tissue diseases in patients from a Portuguese nailfold capillaroscopy clinic. Rheumatology International. 2019;**40**(2):295-301. DOI: 10.1007/s00296-019-04427-0

[51] Cutolo M, Paolino S, Smith V. Nailfold capillaroscopy in rheumatology: Ready for the daily use but with care in terminology. Clinical Rheumatology. 2019;**38**(9):2293-2297. DOI: 10.1007/s10067-019-04716-w

[52] Puechal X, Said G, Hilliquin P, Coste J, Job-Deslandre C, et al. Peripheral neuropathy with necrotizing vasculitis in rheumatoid arthritis. A clinicopathologic and prognostic study of thirty-two patients. Arthritis & Rheumatism. 1995;**38**(11):1618-1629

[53] Makol A, Crowson CS, Wetter DA, Sokumbi O, Matteson EL, Warrington KJ. Vasculitis associated with rheumatoid arthritis: A case-control study. Rheumatology. 2014;**53**:890-899. DOI: 10.1093/rheumatology/ket475

[54] Anwar MM, Tariq E, Khan U, Zaheer M, Ijaz SH. Rheumatoid vasculitis: Is it always a late manifestation of rheumatoid arthritis? Cureus. 2019;**11**(9):e5790. DOI: 10.7759/cureus.5790

[55] Upreti S, Oudah M, Hauptman H, Minn H. Vasculitic neuropathy associated with rheumatoid arthritis, a case report. Journal of Community Hospital Internal Medicine Perspectives. 2019;**9**(5):430-432. DOI: 10.1080/20009666.2019.1676507

[56] Bartels CM, Bridges AJ. Rheumatoid vasculitis: Vanishing menace or target for new treatments? Current Rheumatology Reports.

2010;**12**(6):414-419. DOI: 10.1007/s11926-010-0130-1

[57] Laskaria K, Ahmadi-Simab K, Lamken M, Csernok E, Gross WL, Hellmich B. Are anti-cyclic citrullinated peptide autoantibodies seromarkers for rheumatoid vasculitis in a cohort of patients with systemic vasculitis? Annals of the Rheumatic Diseases. 2010;**69**:469-471

[58] Puéchal X, Gottenberg JE, Berthelot JM, Gossec L, Meyer O, et al. Investigators of the autoimmunity rituximab registry. Rituximab therapy for systemic vasculitis associated with rheumatoid arthritis: Results from the auto immunity and rituximab registry. Arthritis Care and Research. 2012;**64**:331-339

[59] Maher LV, Wilson JG. Successful treatment of rheumatoid vasculitis-associated foot drop with rituximab. Rheumatology. 2006;**45**:1450-1451

Chapter 5

Myopenia and Musculoskeletal Aging in Rheumatoid Arthritis

Dan Xu, Jiake Xu and Lei Dai

Abstract

Rheumatoid arthritis (RA), the commonest inflammatory arthritis, is a debilitating disease leading to decreased functional capacity, social disability and reduced quality of life. RA affects multisystems with chronic inflammatory disease characterized by destructive synovitis and muscular dysfunction leading to premature musculoskeletal aging, which has been coined with many terms including myopenia, sarcopenia, cachexia, muscle failure and muscle wasting. Myopenia is described as the presence of clinically relevant muscle wasting due to any illness at any age, associated with impaired muscle function, increased morbidity and mortality. RA myopenia has significantly less muscle mass compared to the general population muscle loss showing preservation or slight increase in fat mass. RA myopenia is unique compared to chronic disease-related myopenia in cancer, chronic heart failure, kidney disease and chronic infection as it is rarely accompanied by a net weight loss. RA myopenia has younger-age onset compared to elderly primary sarcopenia, while higher-grade inflammation has been considered as the pathophysiology of muscle wasting. Research, however, indicates that inflammation itself cannot fully explain the high prevalence of muscle wasting in RA. This chapter aims to review the literature on the casual relationships among RA myopenia, premature musculoskeletal aging and management strategies to delay musculoskeletal aging.

Keywords: myopenia, rheumatoid arthritis, musculoskeletal aging, chronic inflammation

1. Musculoskeletal aging in the healthy elderly

Muscle mass decreases on advancing age with men losing more absolute and relative muscle mass, especially most prevalent in the seventh decade and beyond [1]. After the age of 50, approximately 1–2% per year of muscle mass is lost, and this age-related reduction in muscle mass and strength is accompanied by intramuscular fat accumulation, muscle atrophy (especially the type IIa fibers), decreased satellite cell proliferation and differentiation capacity, and reduction in motor unit quantity. This muscle remodeling results in changes in muscle architecture that is believed to play a key role in the loss of muscle force and power characteristic of advanced age [2, 3]. Mitchell's group [1] reported only 0.5–1.0% loss of muscle mass per year after 70 and a 4.7% loss compared with peak muscle mass in men and 3.7% decrease for women per decade. Muscle strength simultaneously declines by 10–15% per decade up to 70 years of age, while the muscle strength loss accelerates to between 25 and 40% per decade [4, 5]. Frailty may be regarded as a condition of transition from health to disability during aging. The concept of frailty is often defined as the presence of fatigue, slowness, weakness, low physical activity and exhaustion, which are all mainly related to muscle loss [6].

2. Prevalence of musculoskeletal aging in rheumatoid arthritis

Rheumatoid arthritis (RA) is a chronic inflammatory disease characterized by erosive arthritis and systemic organ involvement with the worldwide prevalence of roughly 5 per 1000 adults. The disease may affect all ages and both sexes; usually, it is seen in young women aged 25–45. The peak incidence is in the sixth decade with recent studies showing that RA is among the most common inflammatory disease in the elderly, accounting for 2% of the geriatric population [7]. The general consensus in the literature is defining rheumatoid arthritis onset after 65 years of age being known as elderly onset RA (EORA). EORA incidence and prevalence in different population-based studies in the world may vary widely, depending on sex and ethnicity [8]. One study showed the incidence rate of RA per 100,000 population over the age of 60 being 9.1 in men and 14.5 in women [9]. A USA study showed the prevalence of RA being 0.5–1%, with 2% in the population over 60 years [10]. The UK-based database Norwalk Arthritis Research (NOAR) showed the incidence of RA increasing with age [11]. The Chinese pooled prevalence showed the estimated population prevalence of RA being 0.37% with 10% elderly onset RA [12]. This fact will likely increase the number of patients with EORA in the coming years to encourage research into the impact of ethnic and geographic differences on the management of RA.

3. Myopenia, sarcopenia, cachexia, muscle failure and muscle wasting disease as one concept in muscle aging of rheumatoid arthritis

3.1 Myopenia and sarcopenia

Myopenia is a relatively new term [13] describing the presence of clinically relevant muscle wasting due to any illness and at any age, associated with clinically relevant degree of muscle wasting, impaired muscle function and increased risks of morbidity or mortality. This term would translate more sufficiently and specifically in clinical settings than sarcopenia, which was introduced in 1988 with the original definition being a "muscle loss" of the appendicular muscle mass in the older people as measured by dual-energy X-ray absorptiometry [14]. In 2010, the European Working Group on Sarcopenia for Older Persons recommended a new operational definition of sarcopenia of aging (primary sarcopenia) including the presence of low muscle mass, low muscle strength and low muscle function and performance [15]. In 2018, two pieces of consensus evidences on sarcopenia of aging were published to combine the update by the European Working Group on Sarcopenia [16] with management of sarcopenia of aging by the International Clinical Practice Guidelines for Sarcopenia [17]. The consensus statement confirms the requirements of low muscle strength (low muscle quality), low muscle mass (low muscle quantity) and muscle functional impairment (low muscle performance) for the clinical diagnosis. Secondary sarcopenia, a similar term to myopenia, is associated with the international consensus definitions specific to malignant sarcopenia in the recent sarcopenia positional review [18]. There are several points of relevance regarding age-related (primary sarcopenia) and disease-related (secondary sarcopenia) loss of muscle mass. Loss of appendicular skeletal muscle mass with aging (primary sarcopenia) occurs continuously in the order of ~5% in men and somewhat lower in women after reaching peak muscle mass in young adulthood at about 30 years of age by a variety of longitudinal observational studies [19, 20]. Another interesting terminology related to secondary sarcopenia is sarcopenic obesity, and the copresence of sarcopenia and obesity has been considered a more deleterious body composition phenotype [21]. In addition to a myriad of cardio-metabolic outcomes related to the effects of fat tissue, higher proportions of fat mass might further affect muscle quality and increase the risk of disability and mortality [22]. A recent Brazil study [23] concluded sarcopenic obesity, but obesity alone was not associated with obstructive sleep apnea (OSA). Both obesity and sarcopenic obesity but not sarcopenia were associated with nocturnal hypoxemia, suggesting a complex pathophysiologic relationship between adverse body composition states and OSA. There are cultural difference in sarcopenic obesity with recent published data of Chinese RA patients, which indicated the lower prevalence of obesity (Chinese 4.2% vs. Westerners 21.4–34.7%) and higher prevalence of underweight (Chinese 17.7% vs. Westerners 1.1–2.2%). Taking together, secondary sarcopenia or myopenia has a non-linear muscle loss curve with a considerably greater magnitude than the linear curve seen in primary sarcopenia. RA patients have significantly less muscle mass compared to the general population, leading to the statement (**Figure 1**) that myopenia is a form of premature disease-related muscular aging in association with connective tissue diseases like rheumatoid arthritis and other chronic diseases shown in **Figure 1**.

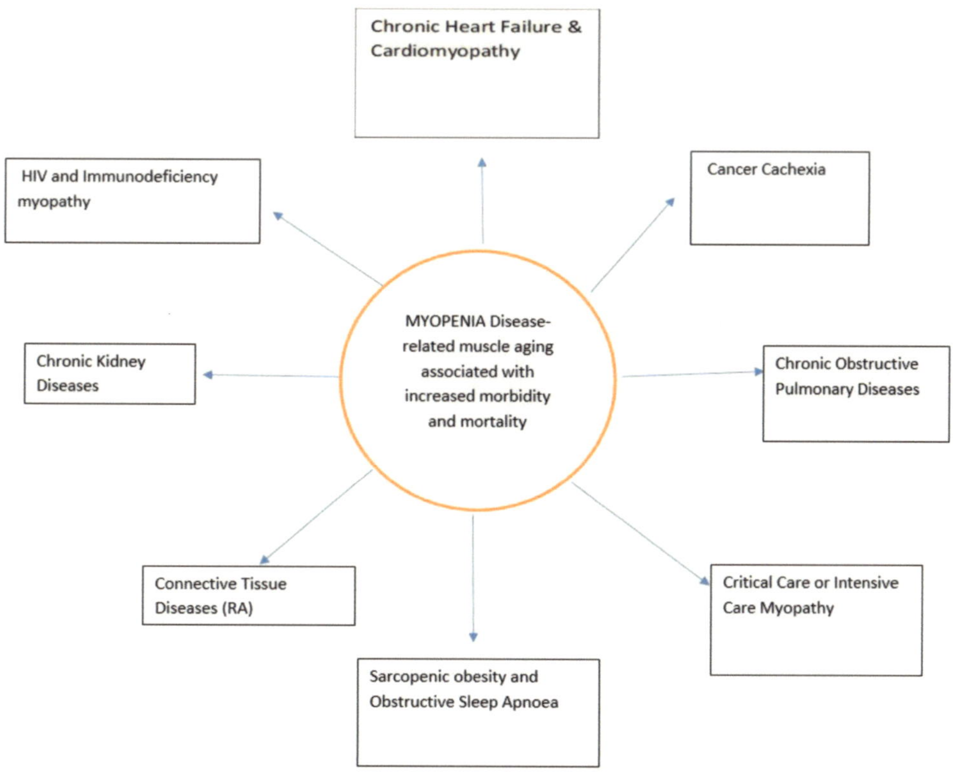

Figure 1.
Myopenia in association with connective tissue diseases like rheumatoid arthritis and other chronic diseases.

3.2 Cachexia, muscle failure and muscle wasting disease

Rheumatoid arthritis cachexia (RAC) is characterized by high degrees of muscle mass loss and muscle strength loss, associated with preservation or slight increase in fat mass [24]. RAC is unique in comparison to other forms of cachexia observed in cancer, chronic heart failure, kidney disease and chronic infection as it is rarely accompanied by a net weight loss [25]. RAC also differs from primary sarcopenia in the elderly as it occurs at much younger age associated with significantly higher muscle mass loss [26]. Higher-grade inflammation has been considered as the central component of the pathophysiology and the key driver of muscle wasting. More recent findings, however, indicate that inflammation on its own cannot fully explain the high prevalence of muscle wasting in RA. Thus, two lifestyle factors including nutrition and physical activity have also been studied to indicate that they play a significant role in muscle wasting in RA, but again neither of these factors seems to be able to fully explain the condition. Oxidative stress is one of the major mechanisms thought to contribute to the development and progression of RA, but its potential contribution to muscle wasting in these patients has received limited attention. Oxidative stress has been shown to promote muscle wasting in healthy populations and people with several chronic conditions. Moreover, all of the aforementioned potential contributors to muscle wasting in RA (i.e., inflammation, nutrition and physical activity) may promote pro- or anti-oxidative mechanisms. Muscle failure is another new term describing the combination of primary and secondary sarcopenia, leading to a more relevant functional definition of premature muscle aging related to rheumatoid arthritis, RA-related muscle failure instead of myopenia. This review will put more emphasis to highlight the important clinical implication of myopenia and premature muscular aging and discuss the various management strategies of delaying musculoskeletal aging in RA, including muscle regeneration *via* reduction in oxidative stress and early control of inflammation via lifestyle and pharmacological interventions.

4. Genetics of RA and muscle aging

RA develops in individuals with a genetic association in RA, which is the presence of DRB1 locus in the HLA class 2 gene. The RA-associated DRB1 alleles share a linear sequence of amino acids between positions 70 and 74 in the HLA-DRB1 chain of the HLA-DRa/b heterodimer, which has led to the 'shared epitope' (SE) hypothesis [27], posing a risk factor for RA development. Jnhi DRB1 allele was associated with early onset of disease, radiological erosion and extra-articular findings [28]. The results of studies investigating genetic predisposition in EORA are inadequate and contradictory [29]. RA-associated DRB1 alleles show differences in early and late onset RA as well as ethnic variants. A Spanish study found that YORA was related to DRB1/04, while EORA was associated with DRB1/01 [30]. This study also found that increased DRB1–13/14 frequency was detected in patients with seronegative EORA and polymyalgia rheumatica (PMR). Another prospective study established the facts that a relationship was found between PMR and DRB1*0101/0102/0401, while seronegative EORA was associated with DRB1-0401. Kim and colleagues investigated the impact of HLA-DRB1 and HLA-DQB1 genes on susceptibility to disease and disease severity in EORA and YORA patients [31]. Alleles encoding the common epitope were detected less frequently in EORA compared with YORA with the effect of the common epitope and HLA-DQ*04 alleles being shown to be less significant. In comparison with YORA, EORA has also been found to have less common epitope presence and less radiological progression.

Hellier and colleagues investigated the effect of the HLA-DRB1 gene on disease susceptibility and disease severity in EORA and YORA [32] and demonstrated HLA-DRB1/04-related alleles were not closely associated in EORA. Thus, it is suggested that the impact of these genes on the susceptibility to disease in EORA is not very important. Wu and colleagues showed that the DRB1/04 allele was detected in half of the EORA population, while the DRB1/04 frequency was 92% in patients with RA starting before 30 years of age [33].

In terms of genetic contribution and impact on the individual variability in muscle aging phenotypes literature on specific gene variants, it remained controversial and no solid evidence exists supporting the existence of an 'unfavorable' genotype associated with accelerated age-related sarcopenia or loss of independent function [34]. Although the ACTN3 R577X polymorphism is the only structural gene for which a clear genotype effect has been shown in human muscle phenotypes, especially for athletic women, there is controversy with regard to which allele (R or X) plays a potential 'favorable' role in aging. The MSTN K153R variation is possibly the strongest candidate to explain variance among muscle phenotypes in the elderly, yet more research is still needed with large cohorts owing to the very low population frequency of the 'unfavorable' 153R allele. Recent evidence [34] indicates that age-related declines in muscle phenotypes are likely polygenic traits and thus not reducible to specific polymorphisms, suggesting that future studies should consider the association between muscle phenotypes in older people including complex gene-gene interactions, interactions between genetic variants that might not influence muscle phenotypes individually and the interaction between genes and chronic disease like rheumatoid arthritis and lifestyle risk factors such as physical activity. It is important to determine those genetic factors that interact with aging and thus modulate functional capacity and genetic predisposition of myopenia in rheumatoid arthritis. It would be also clinically relevant to identify 'unfavorable' genotypes associated with myopenia in rheumatoid arthritis.

5. Pathogenesis of myopenia and musculoskeletal aging in RA

Two major subtypes of RA are classified according to the presence or absence of anti-citrullinated protein antibodies (ACPAs). Citrullination is catalyzed by the calcium-dependent enzyme peptidylarginine deiminase (PAD), changing a positively charged arginine to a polar but neutral citrulline as the result of a post-translational modification. ACPAs can be detected in approximately 67% of RA patients and serve as a useful diagnostic reference for patients with early, undifferentiated arthritis and provide an indication of likely disease progression through to RA [35, 36]. The ACPA-positive subset of RA has a more aggressive clinical phenotype compared to ACPA-negative subset of RA [37]. It is reported that ACPA-negative RA has different genetic association patterns [37] and differential responses of immune cells to citrullinated antigens [38] from those of ACPA-positive subset. In terms of standard treatment [39–41], less effective treatment response of methotrexate (MTX) or rituximab was observed in ACPA-negative subset. Future studies are needed on the potential pathophysiology difference between the two subsets, while this chapter will focus on the ACPA-positive subset of RA and divide the onset and progression of RA process into the above-mentioned EORA and YORA. Since the clinical, genetic and laboratory differences between EORA and YORA are not understood yet, the immunological and hormonal changes in the elderly population may be responsible for the physiological process characterized by reduced T-cell proliferation, reduced antibody synthesis to vaccination and elevated proinflammatory cytokine levels. Immune system changes include T-cell phenotype alteration, reduction in specific immune response, apoptosis defects, cytokine imbalance and inadequate antigen presentation. With increasing age, there is a decrease in the protective immunological response, while the reaction to autoantigens is increasing [42]. In addition, self-tolerance mechanism disorders occur. As a result of thymus involution in senescence, changes in T-cell composition, decrease in T-cell proliferation and cytokine synthesis, as well as decreased antibody synthesis after vaccination, were seen. In one study, elevated interleukin (IL)-6 secretion was associated with dehydroepiandrosterone and androstenedione synthesis in patients with EORA [43]. The acute onset and increased acute phase response seen in EORA may be explained by increased IL-6 levels. Punzi and colleagues showed elevated IL-6 as acute onset and increased acute phase response in the EORA synovial fluid compared with YORA, suggesting the role of IL-6 while no differences were detected in IL-1 and IL-8 levels [44]. Different immunoregulatory mechanisms may be at work in the pathogenesis of RA seen in different age groups with one study by Gamerith and colleagues showing a significantly increased anti-IgG-Fab/free aFab ratio in patients with YORA, compared with EORA, leading to increased rheumatoid factor (RF) presence [45]. Myopenia in RA will be mediated by a similar mechanism of rising IL-6, leading to premature muscle aging in YORA, while acute-onset-induced long-term muscle damage is equivalent to premature muscle aging in EORA. Further research is required to unlock the mechanism of premature muscular aging in RA patients.

6. Clinical features of myopenia in rheumatoid arthritis

Myopenia in rheumatoid arthritis is a similar term to terms described above including secondary sarcopenia, rheumatoid arthritis cachexia and muscle failure or muscle wasting in rheumatoid arthritis. The clinical features follow the two forms of rheumatoid arthritis including EORA and YORA with their distinctive features. EORA has three distinct clinical patterns [46] with the most common clinical form (70%) displaying RF positivity, joint erosions and worse prognosis than YORA, while the second form (25%) is a PMR-like form with proximal limb joint involvement characterized by RF negativity, being associated with acute onset, lack of joint erosions and good prognosis. Non-erosive polyarthritis may be present in 25% of patients with PMR as one of the main differential diagnoses [47]. The presence of metacarpophalangeal (MCP)/proximal interphalangeal (PIP) joint arthritis with proximal limb joint involvement is considered a predictive factor for seronegative EORA. The third EORA pattern is featured by clinical and prognostic similarity to RS3PE syndrome [48] with sudden onset, wrist tenosynovitis, common pitting edema in the hands, HLA-B27 positivity and spontaneous remission within 3–18 months. EORA is not limited to the differentiate diagnosis of PMR, but also associated with other diseases including crystal arthritis, septic arthritis, sarcoidosis and hepatitis C [49]. In many studies [50, 51], simultaneous small and large joint involvement is frequently seen at the onset of the disease, while RF and anti-CCP positivity are seen at similar and/or slightly lower rates in comparison with YORA. Acute onset, PMR-like symptoms, less rheumatoid nodule and RF positivity were detected in EORA compared with YORA. Patients with EORA had a lower joint score and a higher Health Assessment Questionnaire (HAQ) score. A recent study [52] reported the clinical and demographic characteristics of Turkish patients with EORA displaying shoulder joint involvement being more frequent in EORA, while PIP, MCP, elbow and ankle joint involvement were more common in YORA. RA deformities, Sjögren syndrome (SjS) and lung involvement are less common in EORA. Weight loss, myalgia, lymphadenopathy and PMR-like symptoms were also more frequent in EORA, while the antibody profile (RF, ANA, anti-Ro and anti-La) was detected less frequently in EORA. In contrast, anemia of chronic disease, ESR and CRP elevation were more common in a study reported by van der Heijde and colleagues [53]. Another aggressive, destructive EORA form of EORA having more frequent acute onset, initially small and large joint involvement, PMR-like patterns and radiological narrowing of the joint space was reported by Lance and colleagues with radiographic erosive changes [54]. In this report, the patients are characterized by polyarticular small joint involvement, rapid progression, hand/wrist erosions and early hand function loss as well as 63% of these patients reported secondary SjS compared with 25% in patients with YORA. More recently, myopenia has been reported to be very common in Chinese RA patients that is associated with functional limitation and joint damage in RA [55]. In another report at the 2019 American College of Rheumatology meeting, myopenia, equivalent to body composition disorder in elderly Chinese patients with RA, showed that elderly female patients with myopenia were associated with severe joint damage in rheumatoid arthritis [56]. These studies reflected both the cultural and gender diversity of myopenia in RA.

7. Laboratory findings in myopenia in RA

It has been well documented that lower hemoglobin and higher ESR and CRP were detected in EORA in comparison with YORA [57]. In some studies, RF and anti-CCP antibody positivity were reported less frequently in EORA, while in other studies, the frequency of these antibodies was found to be similar in both groups [51, 53, 58]. Chen and colleagues compared the pro-inflammatory cytokine levels of patients with EORA and YORA [59] demonstrating that higher levels of IL-6 and lower levels of tumor necrosis factor α (TNFα) were detected in EORA, associated with higher IL-6 levels being detected in patients with EORA and PMR-like symptoms. Multivariate analysis showed that high IL-1 levels were associated with anti-CCP antibodies, while high TNFα levels were associated with constitutional symptoms in patients with EORA. In comparison with YORA, acute onset, constitutional symptoms and comorbidities were more frequent in patients with EORA.

8. Prognosis of myopenia in RA

There is no direct evidence for discussion with respect to the impact of myopenia on the prognosis of RA. The prognosis of RA in terms of RA's age of onset remains unclear with some studies showing EORA with better prognosis compared with YORA, while others report that they are similar or worse. The above contradictory results may be due to different disease durations between groups examined, bias in patient selection, and different frequencies of seropositivity between younger and older patients. In one study, persistent arthritis was seen in 39% of seropositive patients, while in seronegative patients, this rate was only 6% [60]. In another study, more swollen joints, radiological damage and mortality were reported in seropositive patients in comparison with seronegative patients [61]. In other words, RF and anti-CCP antibodies are considered poor prognostic markers in patients with EORA. Krams and colleagues compared the characteristics of patients with EORA and YORA in the ESPOIR cohort containing 681 patients with RA [62], and the one-year remission rates were higher in the patients with YORA than those with EORA showing more erosion and high HAQ scores in patients with EORA. As a result, at the end of the third year, patients with YORA had higher remission rates, less radiographic progression and lower HAQ scores compared with patients with EORA. A Korean study evaluated 3169 Korean patients with RA [58] and showed that the 486 patients with RA that started when they were over 60 years old were considered to have EORA and it has been found to be an independent risk factor for functional disability. In one study, the presence of acute pitting swelling in the hands at the onset of the disease was shown to be a good prognostic factor [60] with EORA presenting with pitting edema having fewer erosions compared with patients with EORA without pitting edema. In terms of EORA mortality related to myopenia, there was a statistically significant increase in mortality rates in patients with seropositive EORA compared with the general population [57], while there was not significant difference in patients who were seronegative.

9. Treatment and management of myopenia in RA

Management of myopenia in RA will translate the latest research evidence of treatment strategies for rheumatoid arthritis. These strategies include the optimization of lifestyle and risk factor modifications including nutrition and exercise; pharmacological interventions include early administration of disease-modifying antirheumatic drugs (DMARDs); and targeted strategies have been able to prevent radiological progression, reduce morbidity and mortality, and increase functional capacity [63, 64].

10. Exercise and myopenia/cachexia in rheumatoid arthritis

RA and exercise have been thoroughly reviewed [65] to indicate the reduced and compromised exercise capacity in comparison with normal people due to their RA manifestations of pain, stiffness, structural joint damage, bone density loss and muscle weakness [66, 67]. It is well established that physical exercise programs promote prolonged improvements [68] without inducing harmful effects on disease activity and joint damage [69]. Recent evidence [65] has examined different modalities of exercises including resistance training, aerobic training and combination of the two modalities. Aerobic training consists of cycling, aquatics, dancing, walking and running. The final messages show that exercise is effective in reversing joint damage in RA patients as long as RA-specific considerations are being taken into account when developing exercise programs aiming to reduce CVD risk and improve quality of life and maintaining activity of daily living functions of RA patients. In another study [70] describing myopenia/cachexia and exercise types for treatment, intensive progressive resistance training (PRT) can increase lean mass, reduce fat mass, increase strength and improve function. PRT is the most effective exercise to improve skeletal muscle size and strength, even safe when performed at high intensity with RA patients. Resistance training increases tendon stiffness and strengthens connective tissue, while cyclic loading (e.g., walking, cycling and strength endurance exercises) enhances cartilage integrity and joint lubrication as well as mobility exercises increase range of motion. In terms of symptom control in RA patients, exercise can reduce pain and morning stiffness and even reduce fatigue as well as improve functional ability and psychological well-being without exacerbating disease activity. The review also discusses the improvement of patient perceptions regarding the effects and benefits of exercise, clarifies specific exercise recommendations and considers methods of overcoming individual barriers to exercise. A recent study showed that hydrotherapy had a positive role in reducing pain and improving health status of RA patients [71]. All RA patients should be encouraged to include some form of aerobic and resistance exercise training as part of their routine care. More research is still required on the optimal and individualized frequency, intensity, time and types (FITT model) of exercises, or when it requires a combination of types as well as how best to incorporate exercise into the lives of RA patients across the variable course of the disease. Large cohort studies will be required to examine the potential ethnic differences in terms of myopenia and muscle aging in diverse cultures such as in China, India or Africa.

11. Management of frailty and prefrailty in rheumatoid arthritis myopenia

Frailty, which was originally considered a geriatric syndrome [72], is associated with reduced muscle strength, exhaustion and high inflammatory markers [73, 74], leading to perpetuation of the frailty and prefrailty cycle associated with different frailty assessment tools [75, 76]. Frailty and myopenia share a common cardinal clinical feature of reduced muscle strength. A recent study [77] showed that frailty and prefrailty are common in RA patients of younger age and are more prevalent than expected. As the prevalence of frailty increases with age, this study indicates that it is important to counteract frailty for the treatment of myopenia in RA patients. A very interesting aspect for further research would be to assess the frailty status in a large sample size to investigate if the frailty score is lower in RA patients who have entered into permanent remission after early treatment, whereby they did not develop any joint damage, compared to age- and sex-matched patients who have been treated less aggressively.

12. Myopenia, heart failure and premature myocardial aging in RA

RA and other autoimmune chronic inflammatory disorders including psoriasis and inflammatory bowel diseases have been well documented to be associated with considerably increased cardiovascular morbidity and mortality in comparison with the background population [78–82]. In particular, the cardiovascular disease risk in RA patients appears to be comparable with that found in type 2 diabetes mellitus patients [83–85]. Conventional cardiovascular risk factors including hypertension, obesity, dyslipidemia and diabetes mellitus with RA-specific risk factor of increased systemic inflammation have been implicated to contribute significantly [81, 86].

Heart failure (HF), an alternative term describing myopenia in the cardiac muscle, has been shown by numerous public health studies to be associated with increased inflammation and a high prevalence of cardiovascular risk factors [87, 88]. The proinflammatory cytokines of HF promote myocardial damage leading to myopenia of cardiac muscle and other pathogenic manifestations through an array of mechanisms including increased arterial stiffness and endothelial dysfunction [89–95]. A number of review and population studies have examined the risk of developing HF in RA patients and found that RA-specific HF can be independent of cardiovascular risk factors [89, 93, 96, 97]. One of the commonest risk factors and potential cause of HF is ischemic heart disease, which was not shown to be responsible for the increased risks of HF in rheumatoid arthritis. This paper [93] also demonstrated that the increased risks of non-ischemic HF in RA presented early in association with RA severity. A more recent Danish cohort study [98] aimed to investigate the risk of incident HF in RA patients indicated that rheumatoid arthritis was associated with a 30% increased hospitalization for heart failure in comparison with the general population. The clinical Implications of these findings add to the existing evidence that rheumatoid arthritis may be a clinically relevant risk factor for heart failure and premature cardiac muscle aging in RA patients. Future studies examining the value of more extensive screening of RA patients for heart failure are warranted.

In terms of the potential mechanism for increased risks of HF in early course of RA, RA has been associated with left ventricular concentric remodeling and systolic and diastolic left ventricular dysfunction [89, 90, 93, 97]. RA patients are more likely to display significantly elevated levels of circulating cardiac biomarkers including troponins, pro-B-type natriuretic peptides, which are recognized as important prognostic markers of cardiac diseases, especially HF [99]. Thus, it is highly conceivable that chronic systemic inflammation in RA may confer an increased risk of HF and premature myocardial aging that is independent of traditional cardiovascular risk factors.

13. Myopenia and pharmacological intervention in RA

Delaying myopenia and premature muscle aging in RA patients is closely related to the age of onset and preclinical staging of RA. While there are no direct evidences specifically evaluating the impact of pharmacological interventions including synthetic DMARDS and biologics on the management of myopenia in RA, the European League Against Rheumatism guideline advocates early aggressive treatment with these synthetic DMARDS and biologics via their direct effect on reducing inflammation for the purpose of reducing myopenia, delaying premature muscle aging in RA and decreasing cardiovascular morbidity and mortality in RA [100, 101]. These agents are also expected to exert their benefits via their direct effect on reducing inflammation, subsequently improving joint inflammation and function and potentially leading to increased levels of physical activity with consequent reduction of other risk factors including diabetes mellitus and hypertension [100, 101]. A recent study also demonstrates the potential mechanism of how synthetic DMARDS and biologics reduce the risks of sudden cardiac death in RA patients [100].

Identifying a preclinical stage and a growing understanding of the natural history and mechanisms of RA development, alongside new potential pharmacological interventions, shape the prospect that myopenia with premature muscle aging in RA might be preventable in future [102]. The current treatment principles for established RA involve symptomatic management and disease modification. A meta-analysis of 12 published studies confirmed that patients receiving delayed DMARDs therapy were at higher risk of developing radiographic joint space narrowing and bony erosions [103] associated with myopenia in RA with a recent cross-sectional study [55]. In poorly controlled RA patients, bony erosions become more pronounced on radiographs within 2 years of onset and these erosive changes are predictive of poorer functional outcome [104]. In a patient with otherwise unexplained new onset polyarthritis, an urgent referral to a rheumatologist is thus mandatory to confirm an RA diagnosis and early initiation of a DMARDs-based treatment plan aiming for disease remission with delaying myopenia in RA and preventing deformity. Oral corticosteroids are potent and effective anti-inflammatory drugs that may contribute to disease modification [105] to delay myopenia and promote healthy aging. However, this needs to be weighed up against its well-known adverse effects of osteoporosis. Symptomatic management remains the cornerstone interventions throughout the course of the disease with everyday practical measures to deal with the primary symptoms of joint stiffness including pain and fatigue via the mechanism of reducing systemic inflammation. This chapter is not for detailed review and discussion of the pharmacological intervention of RA but endeavors to provide a table from the main author's previous review to summarize the modern pharmacological therapies for RA (**Table 1**) [106].

Classification	Name	Mechanism of action	Potential mechanisms	Side Effect	Reference
Conventional synthetic DMARDs	Methotrexate	Analog of folic acid	Folate-dependent processes; Adenosine signaling; Methyl-donor production; Reactive oxygen species; Adhesion-molecule expression; Cytokine profiles Eicosanoids and MMPs.	Increased liver enzymes, pulmonary damage.	83
	Leflunomide/ Teriflunomide	Pyrimidine synthesis inhibitor	DHODH-dependent pathway; Leukocyte adhesion; Rapidly dividing cells; NF-kB; Kinases; Interleukins; TGF-β.	Hypertension, diarrhea and nausea, hepatotoxicity.	153
	Sulfasalazine	Anti-inflammatory and immunosuppression	Cyclooxygenase and PGE2; Leukotriene production and chemotaxis; Inflammatory cytokines (IL-1, IL-6, TNF-α); Adenosine signaling; NF-kB activation.	Gastrointestinal, central nervous system, and hematologic adverse effect.	154
	Chloroquine /Hydroxychloroquine	Immunomodulatory effects	Toll like receptors; Lysosomotropic action; Monocyte-derived pro-inflammatory cytokines; Anti-inflammatory effects; Cellular immune reactions; T cell responses; Neutrophils; Cartilage metabolism and degradation.	Gastrointestinal tract, skin, central nervous system adverse effect and retinal toxicity.	155
Biological DMARDs					
Antibody-based therapies					
TNF-α targeted therapy	Infliximab	TNF-α inhibitor	Phagocytosis and pro-inflammatory cytokines; Chemoattractant; Adhesion molecules and chemokines; Treg cell function; Function of osteoclasts, leukocytes, endothelial and synovial fibroblasts.	Infection (pneumonia and atypical tuberculosis) injection-site reaction.	
	Adalimumab			Hypertension.	
	Etanercept			Severe /anaphylactoid transfusion reaction.	156
	Golimumab				
	Certolizumab pegol				
B-cell targeted therapy	Rituximab	B cell depleting	Fc receptor gamma-mediated antibody-dependent cytotoxicity and phagocytosis; Complement-mediated cell lysis; antigen presentation; B cell apoptosis; Depletion of CD4+ T cells.	Infection, hypertension, hypogammaglobulinemia, viral reactivation, vaccination responses.	
	Ofatumumab			Late-onset neutropenia.	
	Belimumab	Inhibitors of B cell function		Severe/anaphylactoid transfusion reaction.	157
	Atacicept				
	Tabalumab				
T-cell targeted therapy	Abatacept	CD28/CTLA4 system	Autoantigen recognition; Immune cell infiltrate; T cells activation.	Infection, malignancy.	158
	Belatacept	CD80/CD86			
Interleukin targeted therapy	Tocilizumab	IL-6 inhibition	Innate and the adaptive immune system perturbation; Acute-phase proteins.	Infections (most notably skin and soft tissue), increases in serum cholesterol, transient decreases in neutrophil count and abnormal liver function.	159
	Anakinra	IL-1 inhibition	Inflammatory responses; Matrixenzyme.	Injection site reactions, infections, neutropenia, malignancy.	160
	Canakinumab				
	Rilonacept				
	Secukinumab	IL-17 inhibition	Mitochondrial function; Autophagosome formation.	Infections, nasopharyngitis, candidiasis, neutropenia, safety data of mental health is limited.	161
	Ixekizumab				
Growth and differentiation factors	Denosumab	RANKL inhibitor	Maturation and activation of osteoclast.	Low Ca^{2+} and phosphate in the blood, muscle cramps, cellulitis, and numbness.	162
	Mavrilimumab	GM-CSF inhibitor	Activation, differentiation, and survival of macrophages, dendritic cells, and neutrophils; T helper 1/17 cell; modulation of pain pathways.	Safety file needs further research.	143
Small molecules					
JAK pathway	Tofacitinib	JAK1 and JAK3 inhibitor	T-cell activation, pro-inflammatory cytokine production, synovial inflammation, and structural joint damage.	Zoster infection (advice is to vaccinate beforehand) and other potential side-effects should be monitored carefully through further study.	163, 164
	Baricitinib	JAK1 and JAK2 inhibitor			
	Filgotinib	JAK1 inhibitor			
Future drug and target	Toll like receptors;[165] Bruton's tyrosine kinase;[151] Phosphoinositide-3-kinase pathway;[166] Transforming growth factor-beta;[167] Neuropathways;[168] Dendritic cell[169]				

Table from Ref. [106]. Permission from Bone Research is pending.

Table 1.
Modern pharmacologic therapies for rheumatoid arthritis.

In terms of the age of onset of rheumatoid arthritis, the ultimate goal of RA treatment including EORA and YORA is to control the disease, delay myopenia and maintain functional capacity. As discussed above on genetics, clinical features, pathogenesis and prognosis of EORA and YORA, treatment of EORA should not be so different from treatment of YORA. The goal of treatment should be complete remission or low disease activity based on the principles of treat-to-target strategies. DMARDs used in YORA may also be safely used in the treatment of EORA as long as drug pharmacokinetics and pharmacodynamics in the elderly can be clinically considered with closely monitoring the drug side effect profile [107]. EORA has more comorbid diseases and high number of medications used and consequently increasing drug-drug interactions exacerbating the potential side effect profile [108]. DMARDs used in patients with EORA are limited and contradictory and are receiving less aggressive treatment based on data from patients with EORA in the CORONA database in comparison with those of age- and sex-matched patients with YORA [109]. The study [109] also showed that disease activity and disease severity were similar in both groups. Methotrexate (MTX) use was found to be higher in patients with EORA compared with those with YORA (63.9% vs. 59.6%), while mean MTX dose was found to be higher in patients with YORA. The number of patients using multiple conventional DMARDs or biological DMARDs was found to be lower in those with EORA compared with YORA. Treatment-related toxicity was similar in both groups, whereas toxicity due to MTX was found to be more frequent in the case of YORA. Despite similar disease duration, disease activity and severity, patients with EORA used combined conventional DMARDs and biological DMARDs less frequently compared with patients with YORA. It has been well documented that the age of onset determines the severity of the disease and the choice of treatment [110]. According to Swiss registries, the use of first-line corticosteroids was significantly higher in patients with EORA compared with those with YORA, in contrast to the much lower follow-up on the use of biological drugs [111]. Genevay and colleagues evaluated 1571 patients with RA receiving anti-TNFα drugs [112] and demonstrated similar changes with drug withdrawal rates and mean Disease Activity Score (DAS28) score changes in both groups at the end of the second year. Despite clinical responses, improvement in Health Assessment Questionnaire (HAQ) scores was significantly less in patients with EORA. TNF inhibitors were slightly less or equally effective in reducing disease activity in elderly compared with younger patients with HAQ scores showing less improvement in patients with EORA, especially in patients aged over 75 years [113]. There is limited evidence for the effectiveness of tocilizumab, abatacept, rituximab and tofacitinib in EORA. Tocilizumab was less effective in EORA compared with YORA, while the drug retention rate and discontinuation rates because of adverse events were similar between the two age groups [114]. There is no data on abatacept in EORA, while RCTs showed tofacitinib to be similarly effective in both EORA and YORA [115]. In terms of myopenia in both EORA and YORA, a recent study [116] indicates that EORA is characterized by more equal distribution of sex, higher frequency of acute onset with constitutional symptoms, more frequent involvement of large joints, and lower frequency of RF positivity. Earlier diagnosis, less erosive disease and less DMARD usage were reported as distinguishing patients with EORA from those with YORA. Further studies require the exploration of myopenia and its severity and impact on the prognosis of RA including both EORA and YORA, reflecting the above-mentioned concepts of secondary sarcopenia, cachexia and frailty with old age, potentially impacting RA prognosis in the presence of DMARD side effects.

14. Conclusion and future perspectives

Myopenia and premature muscular aging in RA are similar concepts, raising a lot of research questions in terms of mechanism, lifestyle intervention, comorbidity management and new pharmacological approach. The chapter provides the platform for a discussion about the new term of myopenia and its impact.

Author details

Dan Xu[1,2]*, Jiake Xu[3] and Lei Dai[4]

1 Curtin Medical School, Faculty of Health Sciences, Curtin University, Perth, Australia

2 Department of Medical Education, The First Affiliated Hospital, Sun Yat-Sen University, Guangzhou, Guangdong, China

3 School of Biomedical Sciences, Faculty of Health and Medical Sciences, The University of Western Australia, Perth, Australia

4 Department of Rheumatology, Sun Yat-Sen Memorial Hospital, Sun Yat-Sen University, Guangzhou, Guangdong, China

*Address all correspondence to: daniel.xu@curtin.edu.au

References

[1] Mitchell WK, Williams J, Atherton P, Larvin M, Lund J, Narici M. Sarcopenia, dynapenia, and the impact of advancing age on human skeletal muscle size and strength; a quantitative review. Frontiers in Physiology. 2012;**3**:260

[2] Narici MV, Maffulli N. Sarcopenia: Characteristics, mechanisms and functional significance. British Medical Bulletin. 2010;**95**:139-159

[3] Thomas DR. Loss of skeletal muscle mass in aging: Examining the relationship of starvation, sarcopenia and cachexia. Clinical Nutrition. 2007;**26**(4):389-399

[4] Goodpaster BH, Park SW, Harris TB, et al. The loss of skeletal muscle strength, mass, and quality in older adults: The health, aging and body composition study. The Journals of Gerontology. Series A, Biological Sciences and Medical Sciences. 2006;**61**:1059-1064

[5] Hughes VA, Frontera WR, Wood M, et al. Longitudinal muscle strength changes in older adults: Influence of muscle mass, physical activity, and health. The Journals of Gerontology. Series A, Biological Sciences and Medical Sciences. 2001;**56**:B209-B217

[6] Fried LP, Tangen CM, Walston J, Newman AB, Hirsch C, Gottdiener J, et al. Frailty in older adults: Evidence for a phenotype. The Journals of Gerontology. Series A, Biological Sciences and Medical Sciences. 2001;**56**(3):M146-M156

[7] Laiho K, Tuomilehto J, Tilvis R. Prevalence of rheumatoid arthritis and musculoskeletal diseases in the elderly population. Rheumatology International. 2001;**20**:85-87

[8] Alamanos Y, Voulgari PV, Drosos AA. Incidence and prevalence of rheumatoid arthritis, based on the 1987 ACR criteria: A systematic review. Seminars in Arthritis and Rheumatism. 2006;**36**:182-188

[9] Carbonell J, Cobo T, Descalzo MA, et al. The incidence of rheumatoid arthritis in Spain: Results from a nationwide primary care registry. Rheumatology. 2008;**47**:1088-1092

[10] Rasch EK, Hirsch R, Paulose-Ram R, et al. Prevalence of rheumatoid arthritis in persons 60 years of age and older in the United States. Arthritis & Rheumatology. 2003;**48**:917-926

[11] Symmonds DPM, Barrett EM, Bankhead CR, et al. The incidence of rheumatoid arthritis in the United Kingdom: Results from the Norfolk arthritis register. British Journal of Rheumatology. 1994;**33**:735-739

[12] Xiang YJ, Dai SM. Prevalence of rheumatic diseases and disability in China. Rheumatology International. 2009;**29**:481-490. DOI: 10.1007/s00296-008-0809-z

[13] Fearon K, Evans WJ, Anker SD. Myopenia—A new universal term for muscle wasting. Journal of Cachexia, Sarcopenia and Muscle. 2011;**2**:1-3. DOI: 10.1007/s13539-011-0025-7

[14] Rosenberg IH. Sarcopenia: Origins and clinical relevance. Journal of Nutrition. 1997;**127**(Suppl):990S-991S

[15] Cruz-Jentoft AJ, Baeyens JP, Bauer JM, et al. Sarcopenia: European consensus on definition and diagnosis: Report of the European Working Group on Sarcopenia in Older People. Age and Ageing. 2010;**39**:412-423

[16] Cruz-Jentoft AJ, Bahat G, Bauer J, et al. Sarcopenia: Revised European

consensus on definition and diagnosis. Age and Ageing. 2019;**48**:16-31

[17] Dent E, Morley JE, Cruz-Jentoft AJ, et al. International clinical practice guidelines for sarcopenia (ICFSR): Screening, diagnosis and management. The Journal of Nutrition, Health & Aging. 2018;**22**:1148-1161

[18] Bauer J, Morley JE, Schols AMWJ, Ferrucci L, Cruz-Jentoft AJ, Dent E, et al. Sarcopenia: A time for action. An SCWD position paper journal of cachexia. Sarcopenia and Muscle. 2019;**10**:956-961

[19] Siparsky PN, Kirkendall DT, Garrett WE. Muscle changes in aging: Understanding sarcopenia. Sports Health. 2014;**6**:36-40

[20] Keller K, Engelhardt M. Strength and muscle mass loss with aging process. Age and strength loss. Muscles, Ligaments and Tendons Journal. 2013;**3**(4):346-350

[21] Molino S, Dossena M, Buonocore D, Verri M. Sarcopenic obesity: An appraisal of the current status of knowledge and management in elderly people. The Journal of Nutrition, Health & Aging. 2016;**20**:780-788

[22] Zamboni M, Mazzali G, Fantin F, Rossi A, Di Francesco V. Sarcopenic obesity: A new category of obesity in the elderly. Nutrition, Metabolism, and Cardiovascular Diseases. 2008;**18**:388-395

[23] Piovezan RD, Hirotsu C, Moizinho R, de Sá Souza H, D'Almeida V, Tufik S, et al. Associations between sleep conditions and body composition states: Results of the EPISONO study. Journal of Cachexia, Sarcopenia and Muscle. 2019;**10**:962-973. DOI: 10.1002/jcsm.12445

[24] Roubenoff R, Roubenoff RA, Cannon JG, Kehayias JJ, Zhuang H, Dawson-Hughes B, et al. Rheumatoid cachexia: Cytokine-driven hypermetabolism accompanying reduced body cell mass in chronic inflammation. The Journal of Clinical Investigation. 1994;**93**:2379-2386. DOI: 10.1172/JCI117244

[25] Rajbhadary R, Khezri A, Panush RS. Rheumatoid cachexia: What is it and why is it important? The Journal of Rheumatology. 2011;**38**(3):406-408. DOI: 10.3899/jrheum.101036

[26] Roubenoff R. Rheumatoid cachexia: A complication of rheumatoid arthritis moves into the 21st century. Arthritis Research & Therapy. 2009;**11**:108

[27] Gregersen PK, Silver J, Winchester RJ. The shared epitope hypothesis: An approach to understanding the molecular genetics of susceptibility to rheumatoid arthritis. Arthritis & Rheumatology. 1987;**30**:1205-1213

[28] Mattey DL, Hassell AB, Dawes PT, et al. Independent association of rheumatoid factor and the HLA–DRB1 shared epitope with radiographic outcome in rheumatoid arthritis. Arthritis and Rheumatism. 2001;**44**:1529-1533

[29] Weyand CM, Hicok KC, Conn DL, et al. The influence of HLA–DRB1 genes on disease severity in rheumatoid arthritis. Annals of Internal Medicine. 1992;**117**:801-806

[30] Gonzalez-Gay MA, Hajeer AH, Dababneh A, et al. Sero-negative rheumatoid arthritis in elderly and polymyalgia rheumatica have similar patterns of HLA association. Journal of Rheumatology. 2001;**28**:122-125

[31] Kim EJ, Lee J, Ryu YS, et al. Shared epitope and radiologic progression are less prominent in elderly onset RA than young onset RA. Rheumatology International. 2013;**33**:2135-2140

[32] Hellier JP, Eliaou JF, Daur JP, et al. HLA-DRB1 genes and patients with late onset rheumatoid arthritis. Annals of the Rheumatic Diseases. 2001;**60**:531-533

[33] Wu H, Khanna D, Park G, et al. Interaction between RANKL and HLA-DRB1 genotypes may contribute to younger age at onset of seropositive rheumatoid arthritis in an inception cohort. Arthritis & Rheumatology. 2004;**50**:3093-3103

[34] Garatachea N, Lucía A. Genes and the ageing muscle: A review on genetic association studies. Age. 2013;**35**:207-233. DOI: 10.1007/s11357-011-9327-0

[35] Nishimura K et al. Meta-analysis: Diagnostic accuracy of anti-cyclic citrullinated peptide antibody and rheumatoid factor for rheumatoid arthritis. Annals of Internal Medicine. 2007;**146**:797-808

[36] Bizzaro N et al. Anti-cyclic citrullinated peptide antibody titer predicts time to rheumatoid arthritis onset in patients with undifferentiated arthritis: Results from a 2-year prospective study. Arthritis Research & Therapy. 2013;**15**:R16

[37] Malmstrom V, Catrina AI, Klareskog L. The immunopathogenesis of seropositive rheumatoid arthritis: From triggering to targeting. Nature Reviews. Immunology. 2017;**17**:60-75

[38] Padyukov L et al. A genome-wide association study suggests contrasting associations in ACPA-positive versus ACPA-negative rheumatoid arthritis. Annals of the Rheumatic Diseases. 2011;**70**:259-265

[39] Schuerwegh AJ et al. Evidence for a functional role of IgE anticitrullinated protein antibodies in rheumatoid arthritis. Proceedings of the National Academy of Sciences of the United States of America. 2010;**107**:2586-2591

[40] van Dongen H et al. Efficacy of methotrexate treatment in patients with probable rheumatoid arthritis: A double-blind, randomized, placebo-controlled trial. Arthritis and Rheumatism. 2007;**56**:1424-1432

[41] Sellam J et al. B cell activation biomarkers as predictive factors for the response to rituximab in rheumatoid arthritis: A six-month, national, multicenter, open-label study. Arthritis and Rheumatism. 2011;**63**:933-938

[42] Seegobin SD et al. ACPA-positive and ACPA-negative rheumatoid arthritis differ in their requirements for combination DMARDs and corticosteroids: Secondary analysis of a randomized controlled trial. Arthritis Research & Therapy. 2014;**16**:R13

[43] Raychaudhuri S et al. Five amino acids in three HLA proteins explain most of the association between MHC and seropositive rheumatoid arthritis. Nature Genetics. 2012;**44**:291-296

[44] Okada Y et al. Risk for ACPA-positive rheumatoid arthritis is driven by shared HLA amino acid polymorphisms in Asian and European populations. Human Molecular Genetics. 2014;**23**:6916-6926

[45] Mori M, Yamada R, Kobayashi K, Kawaida R, Yamamoto K. Ethnic differences in allele frequency of autoimmune-disease-associated SNPs. Journal of Human Genetics. 2005;**50**:264-266

[46] Healey LA. Subsets of rheumatoid arthritis in the aged. Arthritis & Rheumatology. 1986;**29**:149

[47] Healey LA, Sheets PK. The relation of polymyalgia rheumatica to rheumatoid arthritis. Journal of Rheumatology. 1988;**15**:750-752

[48] McCartey DJ, O'Duffy JD, Pearson L, et al. Remitting seronegative

symmetrical synovitis with pitting edema. JAMA. 1985;**254**:2763-2767

[49] Inoue K, Shichikawa K, Nishioka J, et al. Older age onset rheumatoid arthritis with or without osteoarthritis. Annals of the Rheumatic Diseases. 1987;**46**:908-911

[50] Goemaere S, Ackerman C, Goethals K, et al. Onset of symptoms of rheumatoid arthritis in relation to age, sex and menopausal transition. Journal of Rheumatology. 1990;**17**:1620-1622

[51] Ferraccioli GF, Cavalieri F, Mercandati M, et al. Clinical features, scintiscan characteristics and X-ray progression of late onset rheumatoid arthritis. Clinical and Experimental Rheumatology. 1984;**2**:157-161

[52] Türkçapar N, Demir O, Atli T, et al. Late onset rheumatoid arthritis: Clinical and laboratory comparisons with younger onset patients. Archives of Gerontology and Geriatrics. 2006;**42**:225-231

[53] van der Heijde DM, van Riel PL, van Leeuwen MA, et al. Older versus younger onset rheumatoid arthritis: Results at onset and after 2 years of a prospective follow-up study of early rheumatoid arthritis. Journal of Rheumatology. 1991;**18**:1285-1289

[54] Lance NJ, Curran JJ. Late-onset, seropositive, erosive rheumatoid arthritis. Seminars in Arthritis and Rheumatism. 1993;**23**:177-182

[55] Lin JZ, Liang JJ, Ma JD, Li QH, Mo YQ, Cheng WM, et al. Myopenia is associated with joint damage in rheumatoid arthritis: A cross-sectional study. Journal of Cachexia, Sarcopenia and Muscle. 2019;**10**:355-367. DOI: 10.1002/jcsm.12381

[56] Chen CT, Lin JZ, Ma JD, Li QH, Mo YQ, Chen LF, et al. Myopenia in elderly female patients with rheumatoid arthritis is associated with severe joint damage: A cross-sectional study. In: 2019 ACR/ARP Annual Meeting Abstract 475

[57] van Schaardenburg D, Hazes JM, de Boer A, et al. Outcome of rheumatoid arthritis in relation to age and rheumatoid factor at diagnosis. Journal of Rheumatology. 1993;**20**:45-52

[58] Cho SK, Sung YK, Choi CB, et al. Do patients with elderly-onset rheumatoid arthritis have severe functional disability? Seminars in Arthritis and Rheumatism. 2012;**42**:23-31

[59] Chen DY, Hsieh TY, Chen YM, et al. Proinflammatory cytokine profiles of patients with elderly-onset rheumatoid arthritis: A comparison with younger-onset disease. Gerontology. 2009;**55**:250-258

[60] Pease CT, Bhakta BB, Devlin J, et al. Does the age of onset of rheumatoid arthritis influence phenotype? A prospective study of outcome and prognostic factors. Rheumatology (Oxford). 1999;**38**:228-234

[61] Calvo-Alen J, Corrales A, Sanchez-Andrada S, et al. Outcome of late-onset rheumatoid arthritis. Clinical Rheumatology. 2005;**24**:485-489

[62] Krams T, Ruyssen-Witrand A, Nigon D, et al. Effect of age at rheumatoid arthritis onset on clinical, radiographic, and functional outcomes: The ESPOIR cohort. Joint, Bone, Spine. 2016;**83**:511-515

[63] Wabe N, Wiese MD. Treating rheumatoid arthritis to target: Physician and patient adherence issues in contemporary rheumatoid arthritis therapy. Journal of Evaluation in Clinical Practice. 2017;**23**:486-493

[64] Aletah D, Smolen JS. Diagnosis and management of rheumatoid arthritis: A review. JAMA. 2018;**320**(13)

[65] Metsios GS, Stavropoulos-Kalinoglou A, Veldhuijzen van Zanten JJCS, Treharne GJ, Panoulas VF, Douglas KMJ, et al. Rheumatoid arthritis, cardiovascular disease and physical exercise: A systematic review. Rheumatology. 2008;**47**:239-248. DOI: 10.1093/rheumatology/kem260

[66] Lee DM, Weinblatt ME. Rheumatoid arthritis. Lancet. 2001;**358**:903-911

[67] Ekdahl C, Broman G. Muscle strength, endurance, and aerobic capacity in rheumatoid arthritis: A comparative study with healthy subjects. Annals of the Rheumatic Diseases. 1992;**51**:35-40

[68] de Jong Z, Munneke M, Zwinderman AH, et al. Is a long-term high-intensity exercise program effective and safe in patients with rheumatoid arthritis? Results of a randomized controlled trial. Arthritis and Rheumatism. 2003;**48**:2415-2424

[69] Hakkinen A. Effectiveness and safety of strength training in rheumatoid arthritis. Current Opinion in Rheumatology. 2004;**16**:132-137

[70] Cooney JK, Law R-J, Matschke V, Lemmey AB, Moore JP, Ahmad Y, et al. Benefits of exercise in rheumatoid arthritis. Journal of Aging Research. 2011; Article ID 681640, 14 p. DOI: 10.4061/2011/681640

[71] Al-Qubaeissy KY, Fatoye FA, Goodwin PC, et al. The effectiveness of hydrotherapy in the Management of Rheumatoid Arthritis: A systematic review Musculoskelet. Care. 2013;**11**:3-18

[72] Fried LP, Ferrucci L, Darer J, Williamson JD, Anderson G. Untangling the concepts of disability, frailty, and comorbidity: Implications for improved targeting and care. The Journals of Gerontology. Series A, Biological Sciences and Medical Sciences. 2004;**59**:25563

[73] Espinoza SE, Fried LP. Risk factors for frailty in the older adult. Clinical Geriatrics. 2007;**15**:37-44

[74] Yao X, Li H, Leng SX. Inflammation and immune system alterations in frailty. Clinics in Geriatric Medicine. 2011;**27**:79-87

[75] Dent E, Kowal P, Hoogendijk EO. Frailty measurement in research and clinical practice: A review. European Journal of Internal Medicine. 2016;**31**:3-10

[76] De Vries NM, Staal JB, van Ravensberg CD, Hobbelen JS, Olde Rikkert MG, Nijhuis-van Der Sanden MW. Outcome instruments to measure frailty: A systematic review. Ageing Research Reviews. 2011;**10**:104-114

[77] Haider S, Grabovac I, Berner C, Lamprecht T, Fenzl K-H, Erlacher L, et al. Frailty in seropositive rheumatoid arthritis patients of working age: A cross-sectional. Clinical and Experimental Rheumatology. 2019;**37**:585-592

[78] Armstrong EJ, Harskamp CT, Armstrong AW. Psoriasis and major adverse cardiovascular events: A systematic review and meta-analysis of observational studies. Journal of the American Heart Association. 2013;**2**:e000062. DOI: 10.1161/JAHA.113.000062

[79] Avina-Zubieta JA, Thomas J, Sadatsafavi M, Lehman AJ, Lacaille D. Risk of incident cardiovascular events in patients with rheumatoid arthritis: A meta-analysis of observational studies.

Annals of the Rheumatic Diseases. 2012;**71**:1524-1529

[80] Filimon AM, Negreanu L, Doca M, Ciobanu A, Preda CM, Vinereanu D. Cardiovascular involvement in inflammatory bowel disease: Dangerous liaisons. World Journal of Gastroenterology. 2015;**21**:9688-9692

[81] Soubrier M, Barber Chamoux N, Tatar Z, Couderc M, Dubost JJ, Mathieu S. Cardiovascular risk in rheumatoid arthritis. Joint, Bone, Spine. 2014;**81**:298-302

[82] Ahlehoff O, Gislason GH, Charlot M, Jorgensen CH, Lindhardsen J, Olesen JB, et al. Psoriasis is associated with clinically significant cardiovascular risk: A Danish nationwide cohort study. Journal of Internal Medicine. 2011;**270**:147-157

[83] Brady SR, de Courten B, Reid CM, Cicuttini FM, de Courten MP, Liew D. The role of traditional cardiovascular risk factors among patients with rheumatoid arthritis. The Journal of Rheumatology. 2009;**36**:34-40

[84] Lindhardsen J, Ahlehoff O, Gislason GH, Madsen OR, Olesen JB, Torp-Pedersen C, et al. The risk of myocardial infarction in rheumatoid arthritis and diabetes mellitus: A Danish nationwide cohort study. Annals of the Rheumatic Diseases. 2011;**70**(6):929-934. DOI: 10.1136/ard.2010.143396

[85] Peters MJ, van Halm VP, Voskuyl AE, Smulders YM, Boers M, Lems WF, et al. Does rheumatoid arthritis equal diabetes mellitus as an independent risk factor for cardiovascular disease? A prospective study. Arthritis and Rheumatism. 2009;**61**:1571-1579

[86] del Rincon I, Polak JF, O'Leary DH, Battafarano DF, Erikson JM, Restrepo JF, et al. Systemic inflammation and cardiovascular risk factors predict rapid progression of atherosclerosis in rheumatoid arthritis. Annals of the Rheumatic Diseases. 2015;**74**:1118-1123

[87] Go AS, Mozaffarian D, Roger VL, Benjamin EJ, Berry JD, Borden WB. Heart disease and stroke statistics—2013 update: A report from the American Heart Association. Circulation. 2013;**127**:e6-e245

[88] Kalogeropoulos A, Georgiopoulou V, Psaty BM, Rodondi N, Smith AL, Harrison DG, et al. Inflammatory markers and incident heart failure risk in older adults: The health ABC (health, aging, and body composition) study. Journal of the American College of Cardiology. 2010;**55**:2129-2137

[89] Aslam F, Bandeali SJ, Khan NA, Alam M. Diastolic dysfunction in rheumatoid arthritis: A meta-analysis and systematic review. Arthritis Care and Research. 2013;**65**:534-543

[90] Cioffi G, Viapiana O, Ognibeni F, Dalbeni A, Giollo A, Gatti D, et al. Prognostic role of subclinical left ventricular systolic dysfunction evaluated by speckle-tracking echocardiography in rheumatoid arthritis. Journal of the American Society of Echocardiography. 2017;**30**:602-611

[91] Foster W, Carruthers D, Lip GY, Blann AD. Inflammation and microvascular and macrovascular endothelial dysfunction in rheumatoid arthritis: Effect of treatment. The Journal of Rheumatology. 2010;**37**:711-716

[92] Marti CN, Gheorghiade M, Kalogeropoulos AP, Georgiopoulou VV, Quyyumi AA, Butler J. Endothelial dysfunction, arterial stiffness, and heart failure. Journal of the American College of Cardiology. 2012;**60**:1455-1469

[93] Midtbo H, Semb AG, Matre K, Kvien TK, Gerdts E. Disease activity is associated with reduced left ventricular systolic myocardial function in patients with rheumatoid arthritis. Annals of the Rheumatic Diseases. 2017;**76**:371-376

[94] Paulus WJ, Tschope C. A novel paradigm for heart failure with preserved ejection fraction: Comorbidities drive myocardial dysfunction and remodeling through coronary microvascular endothelial inflammation. Journal of the American College of Cardiology. 2013;**62**:263-271

[95] Fan F, Galvin A, Fang L, White DA, Moore XL, Sparrow M, et al. Comparison of inflammation, arterial stiffness and traditional cardiovascular risk factors between rheumatoid arthritis and inflammatory bowel disease. Journal of Inflammation (London). 2014;**11**:29

[96] Mantel A, Holmqvist M, Andersson DC, Lund LH, Askling J. Associationbetweenrheumatoidarthritis and risk of ischemic and nonischemic heart failure. Journal of the American College of Cardiology. 2017;**69**:1275-1285

[97] Nicola PJ, Maradit-Kremers H, Roger VL, Jacobsen SJ, Crowson CS, Ballman KV, et al. The risk of congestive heart failure in rheumatoid arthritis: A population-based study over 46 years. Arthritis and Rheumatism. 2005;**52**:412-420

[98] Khalid U, Egeberg A, Ahlehoff O, Lane D, Gislason GH, Lip GYH, et al. Incident heart failure in patients with rheumatoid arthritis: A nationwide cohort study. Journal of the American Heart Association. 2018;**7**:e007227. DOI: 10.1161/JAHA.117.007227

[99] Avouac J, Meune C, Chenevier-Gobeaux C, Dieude P, Borderie D, Lefevre G, et al. Inflammation and disease activity are associated with high circulating cardiac markers in rheumatoid arthritis independently of traditional cardiovascular risk factors. The Journal of Rheumatology. 2014;**41**:248-255

[100] Masoud S, Lim PB, Kitas GD, Panoulas V. Sudden cardiac death in patients with rheumatoid arthritis. World Journal of Cardiology. 2017;**9**(7):562-573

[101] Peters MJ, Symmons DP, McCarey D, Dijkmans BA, Nicola P, Kvien TK, et al. EULAR evidence-based recommendations for cardiovascular risk management in patients with rheumatoid arthritis and other forms of inflammatory arthritis. Annals of the Rheumatic Diseases. 2010;**69**:325-331. DOI: 10.1136/ard.2009.113696

[102] Deane KD. Can rheumatoid arthritis be prevented? Best Practice & Research. Clinical Rheumatology. 2013;**27**:467-485

[103] Finckh A, Liang MH, van Herckenrode CM, de Pablo P. Long-term impact of early treatment on radiographic progression in rheumatoid arthritis: A metaanalysis. Arthritis and Rheumatism. 2006;**55**:864-872

[104] Fuchs HA, Kaye JJ, Callahan LF, Nance EP, Pincus T. Evidence of significant radiographic damage in rheumatoid arthritis within the first 2 years of disease. The Journal of Rheumatology. 1989;**16**:585-591

[105] Cohen S, Emery P. The American College of Rheumatology/European League Against Rheumatism criteria for the classification of rheumatoid arthritis: A game changer. Arthritis and Rheumatism. 2010;**62**:2592-2594

[106] Guo X, Wang Y, Xu D, Nossent J, Pavlos NJ, Xu J. Rheumatoid arthritis: Pathological mechanisms and modern pharmacologic therapies. Bone

Research. 2018;**6**:15. DOI: 10.1038/s41413-018-0016-9

[107] Studenski SA, Ward MM. Pharmacology and the elderly. In: Harris ED Jr, Budd RC, Firestein GS, et al., editors. Kelley's Textbook of Rheumatology. 7th ed. Philadelphia, PA: Elsevier Saunders; 2005. pp. 961-966

[108] Walker J, Wynne H. The frequency and severity of adverse drug reactions in older people. Age and Ageing. 1994;**23**:255-259

[109] Tutuncu Z, Reed G, Kremer J, et al. Do patients with older-onset rheumatoid arthritis receive less aggressive treatment? Annals of the Rheumatic Diseases. 2006;**65**:1226-1229

[110] Innala L, Berglin E, Moler B, et al. Age at onset determines severity and choice of treatment in early rheumatoid arthritis: A prospective study. Arthritis Research & Therapy. 2014;**16**:R94

[111] Mueller RB, Reshiti N, Kaegi T, et al. Does addition of glucocorticoids to the initial therapy influence the later course of the disease in patients with early RA? Results from the Swiss prospective observational registry (SCQM). Clinical Rheumatology. 2017;**36**:59-66

[112] Genevay S, Finckh A, Ciurea A, et al. Tolerance and effectiveness of anti-tumor necrosis-alpha therapies in elderly patients with rheumatoid arthritis: A population based cohort study. Arthritis and Rheumatism. 2007;**57**:679-685

[113] Bathon JM, Fleischmann RM, Van der Heijde D, et al. Safety and efficacy of etanercept treatment in elderly subjects with rheumatoid arthritis. The Journal of Rheumatology. 2006;**33**:234-243

[114] Pers YM, Schaub R, Constant E, et al. Efficacy and safety of tocilizumab in elderly patients with rheumatoid arthritis. Joint, Bone, Spine. 2015;**82**:25-30

[115] Curtis JR, Schulze-Koops H, Takiya L, et al. Efficacy and safety of tofacitinib in older and younger patients with rheumatoid arthritis. Annals of the Rheumatic Diseases. 2013;**65** (Suppl 10):2331

[116] Kobak S, Bes C. An autumn tale: Geriatric rheumatoid arthritis. Therapeutic Advances in Musculoskeletal Disease. 2018;**10**(1):3-11

Section 4

Medical and Patient Self Management Programs in Rheumatoid Arthritis

Chapter 6

Diagnostic Challenges and Management Update in Rheumatoid Arthritis

Mihail Virgil Boldeanu, Adrian Răzvan Ionescu, Valeriu Horațiu Popoviciu, Andreea Lili Bărbulescu, Ștefan Cristian Dinescu, Isabela Siloși, Maria Forțofoiu, Rodica Pădureanu, Andreea Meca, Vlad Pădureanu, Mircea Cătălin Forțofoiu, Ioan Sabin Poenariu, Lidia Boldeanu and Ananu Florentin Vreju

Abstract

Rheumatoid arthritis is a chronic, systemic inflammatory disease, with certain evidence of multiple factors involved, but also with the strong autoimmune component, leading to a high potential for disability, through synovial inflammation and joint destruction. Diagnostic methods and management possibilities have recently improved, thus leading to a better outcome, based on the treat to target recommendation. Although biologic agents represent efficient therapeutic agents, in the last few years, the advances in understanding the mediators involved in rheumatoid arthritis pathogenesis have provided new targeted therapies, represented by small molecule inhibitors against the Janus kinases that contribute in the signaling pathways of various cytokine receptors.

Keywords: rheumatoid arthritis, autoimmune disease, biologic agents, new therapies

1. Introduction

Rheumatoid arthritis (RA) is a chronic, autoimmune, systemic disease that targets primarily the synovial joint lining and causes progressive disability. Untreated, PR leads to the destruction of the joints by the erosion of cartilage and bone material. Loss of physical function is the aftermath, which is why early treatment is vital for controlling disease activity and for preventing joint damage.

Angiogenesis is an important process for the growth and development of all tissues, during which new blood vessels are formed from pre-existing vascularization and play a critical role in the pathogenesis of several inflammatory autoimmune diseases, such as PR. Angiogenesis is triggered by the dominance of pro-angiogenic factors over endogenous angiostatic mediators. Studies conducted over the past two decades have suggested the involvement of numerous pro-angiogenic factors such as metabolites, ions, growth factors, hypoxia-inducible factors, cytokines, chemokines, extracellular matrix metalloproteinases, and adhesion molecules, in RA pathogenesis.

Also, these pro-angiogenic factors were targets for possible therapies. Thus, the research has led to the emergence of new therapies with a key role in modulating the activity of the cellular immune response and inflammation in the synovial tissue.

According to studies, patients with RA, after treatment with biological agents, showed a significant decrease compared to the initial levels of acute-phase reactants and inflammatory proteins: C-reactive protein (CRP), the red blood cells sedimentation rate (ESR), pro-inflammatory cytokines (tumor necrosis factor-alpha, TNF-α; interleukins, IL-17, IL-8, IL-18), chemokines (CXCL12), growth factors (angiopoietins, Ang-1, Ang-2; growth factor of vascular endothelium, VEGF), adhesion molecules (vascular adhesion molecule 1, VCAM-1) and matrix metalloproteinases (MMP-9 and MMP-13).

Biological therapy has brought many benefits for patients, by improving the prognosis, evolution, stopping or reducing destructive lesions, obtaining remission and thus increasing the quality of life and maintaining social integration.

Biological therapy is no longer reserved only for cases that do not respond to classical therapy, as clinical studies have shown that the number of swollen and painful joints decreases, as well as the rate of osteoarticular destructive lesions.

2. Rheumatoid arthritis: pathogenesis

The pathological mechanisms that drive the synovial inflammation and structural damage in RA are complex.

Research in the field of RA pathogenesis has been an essential tool in the development of disease-modifying drugs, biologic therapy, and the more recent targeted therapy. There are separate domains of research that combine to offer a complete picture of the disease etiopathogenesis. These include the study of trigger agents, autoantigen-autoantibody interaction, genetic susceptibility, articular and extraarticular pathology. Major disease subtypes defined by anti-citrulline peptide antibody (ACPA) positivity provide some differences in genetic associations, immune response, disease severity and treatment effectiveness [1].

The presence of ACPA is highly specific for RA [2] and occurs in response to a set of citrullinated proteins, such as fibrin, fibronectin, vimentin, type II collagen and histones [3]. Citrullination is catalyzed by peptidylarginine-deiminase (PAD), a calcium-dependent enzyme. Another post-translational process that drives the formation of autoantigen in RA is carbamylation. It is defined by the change of the amino acid lysine to homocitrulline. Smoking and chronic inflammation, both characteristic features in the context of RA pathogenesis, are thought to enhance the process of carbamylation [4].

A series of environmental factors, such as cigarette smoking and silica have been associated with RA development. Smoking has provided some strong evidence of the potential to generate citrullinated proteins. In a historical Danish twin cohort study, Svendsen et al. concluded that 20 years of smoking doubles the risk of RA development [5]. Environmental factors can generate an epigenetic regulation and influence specific RA immune reactions to citrullinated proteins [6]. Exposure to smoke, silica or carbon-derived nanomaterials can activate antigen-presenting cells and PADs by triggering mucosal toll-like receptors.

Pathogenic infections associated with the onset of rheumatoid arthritis can lead to a faulty immunological tolerance towards essential self-antigens. This can subsequently cause chronic joint inflammation along with an imbalance between the various T helper subsets [7].

Among the infectious agents regarded as potential triggering factors, *Porphyromonas gingivalis* and *Aggregatibacter actinomycetemcomitans* are of particular interest. Studies on both microorganisms have linked periodontal infection to RA autoimmunity. *P. gingivalis* is constitutively equipped with the PAD enzyme [8]. The presence of *P. gingivalis* has been linked to both autoantigen release and ACPA production [3]. Periodontal space and lungs are thus considered potential triggering sites for RA. The role of *Epstein–Barr virus* (EBV), *cytomegalovirus* and *parvovirus B19* (B19) are controversial. Sherina et al. conclude in a 2017 study that high antiviral antibody levels for EBV and B19 may, in fact, have a protective role against ACPA-positive RA [9].

When highlighting the etiopathogenesis of RA, certain species of *Collinsella* are involved by establishing an increase in gut permeability, a decrease in the activity of tight junction proteins and by way of regulating the synthesis of IL-17A at the level of the epithelium. More broadly, gut dysbiosis has been implicated in the pathogenesis of RA through the recruitment of essential inflammatory mediators such as TNF-alfa, IL-6, and IL-17A [10]. One metagenome-wide association study recently revealed a link between RA and multiple species belonging to the genus *Prevotella,* such as *Prevotella denticola* [11].

There has not been thus far sufficient evidence to advocate for a clinical correlation between an infection with *Helicobacter pylori* (*H. pylori*) and RA, despite the results of experiments performed in vitro, which have revealed that chronic stimulation of B lymphocytes with the urease made by the *H. pylori* leads to an increased production of autoantibodies, specifically rheumatoid factor (RF), an immunoglobulin M (IgM) antibody directed to the Fc portion of IgG. While RA patients are at risk of developing peptic ulcers, it is unclear whether this is due to an increased prevalence of *H. pylori* infection or because of the ample use of anti-inflammatory, non-steroidal medication [12].

It is known that viruses can modify the clinical picture depending on genetic background, immune responses elicited by the host and the type of virus strain involved. Certain viruses such as *parainfluenza* have been associated with a higher incidence of RA in men, and more broadly with both male and female patients below the age of 40 [13].

There is an overall agreement that pathogenesis in RA is linked with genetic susceptibility. Studies have found more than 100 susceptibility loci in RA patients [14]. Twin studies in which heritability is reported to be ~60% provides strong evidence for this matter. It is also speculated that the interplay between environmental factors and genetics may, in fact, lay the foreground for the specific autoimmune reactions and further transition to the joint disease stage. A major genetic risk factor associated with RA concerns the human leucocyte antigen (HLA) class II region. The conserved amino acid sequence located at the antigen-binding site of the antigen-presenting molecule, encoded by the alleles of HLA-DRB1 is referred to as the shared epitope (SE) [14]. The strongest genetic associations in RA are identified in the HLA-DR1 and HLA-DR4 serotypes. Some studies do not link the HLA II locus to ACPA response directly [15, 16], rather to the progression from ACPA(+) to ACPA(+) RA, through a process of maturation via T cells which activate ACPA-producing B-cells. It is assumed that SEs play an important role in the antigen presentation process. Thus the different alleles at the SE level can influence the interaction between HLA class-II and the specific receptor of T lymphocytes (TCR) or between HLA class-II and antigen. Studies on SE phenotypes and specific HLA-DRB1 subtypes revealed that HLA-DRB1*04 has a significantly higher frequency in RA and is associated with seropositivity independent of the smoking status [17, 18].

ACPA(+) and ACPA(−) RA patients have similar hereditability, reported at 68% and 66%, respectively. The two serotypes display differences in genetic susceptibility, including a significantly lower SE contribution in the seronegative disease of 2.4%, compared to 18% in ACPA(+) RA [19]. A major genetic risk factor outside the HLA region concerns the protein tyrosine phosphatase non-receptor 22 (PTPN22) gene [14]. Other non-HLA susceptibility genes identified in both disease subgroups include TNFAIP3, GIN1/C5orf30, STAT4, ANKRD55/IL6ST, BLK [14]. The protective role of specific HLA-DRB1 alleles has been reported in one meta-analysis, in which HLA-DRB1*13 accounted for a lower risk of ACPA-positive RA [20]. Studies on the outcome of patients with undifferentiated arthritis determined several susceptibility loci (PTPN22, TRAF1/C5, AFF3, KIF5A, TAGAP) related to disease severity [21]. These genetic loci may provide a tipping point in the disease progression and identify as prognosis markers for the transition to an established RA [14].

Autoantibody secretion generated by the autoantigen release can precede the onset of fulminant joint disease by several years [22]. High-titer RF is of high diagnostic and prognostic value and is linked to erosive RA. ACPA is the most specific marker antibodies for RA and is linked, similarly to RF with erosive disease. Another autoantigen with potential pathogenetic relevance is the heterogeneous nuclear ribonucleoprotein-A2 (RA33) which is targeted by autoreactive T cells [2].

Both the innate and adaptive immune systems contribute to initial antibody production and further development of sustained chronic synovitis. The fibroblast-like synoviocytes interact with cells of the innate immune system which include macrophages, monocytes, mast cells, and dendritic cells. ACPA target citrullinated proteins on the surface of macrophages and monocytes, which in turn enhances the production of pro-inflammatory mediators [3]. Activated mast cells have an essential contribution to the pro-inflammatory milieu through IL-17 A secretion [23]. The involvement of the adaptive immune response is based on the antigen activation of major histocompatibility complex (MHC) class II dependent on T cells (cell-mediated immunity), cytokine release, and stimulation of B-cell antibody production (humoral immunity).

The exact relationship between reported antibodies relating to the disease and the pathogenic features observed remains a mystery due to lack of research. Limited data thus far comparing RA serotypes indicate different underlying processes that can drive parallel pathways towards similar clinical phenotypes. There is evidence of T-cell-mediated immune dysregulation in RA irrespective of autoantibody production [24]. Serotype distinctions include differences in immune cells subtypes, cytokines and chemokines [25].

The synovium in patients with established RA displays an inflammatory infiltrate composed of a heterogeneous set of immune cells. Neutrophils present in the synovial fluid have an extended lifespan and feature an enhanced production of reactive oxygen species and neutrophil extracellular traps (NETosis) [25]. Synovial T cells, especially CD28-CD4+ T cells are autoreactive, produce interferon-gamma (IFN-γ) and are resistant to apoptosis [26]. Differentiated effector T cells, helper types (Th1, Th2, Th17) contribute to cytokine secretion. Antigen-specific T cells or T cells activated by the pro-inflammatory milieu of the synovia are capable of stimulating monokine production by monocytes and macrophage-like synoviocytes, especially interleukins (IL-1, IL-6) and TNF-α [26]. The T-cell dependent IL-17 cytokine has a significant pathogenic role by inducing cartilage degradation and bone erosion through stimulation of receptor activator of NF-κB ligand expression on osteoblasts. The Th17 cells population is increased both in joints and peripheral blood of patients with RA [27]. IL-23 produced by dendritic cells promotes the survival and expansion of Th17 cells. It is thought that an imbalance between IL-12 (Th17 inhibitor) and IL-23 secretion by dendritic cells contributes to RA pathogenesis [26].

Various chemokines, cytokines, growth factors, and cell adhesion molecules promote neovascularization in the setting of chronic inflammation. In RA, there is an abundance of angiogenic factors, of which VEGF is of major importance. Inflammatory cytokines, such as TNF-α, IL-1, IL-6, IL-17, IL-18, granulocyte and granulocyte-macrophage colony-stimulating factors (GM-CSF), may also induce angiogenesis through VEGF-dependent pathway [28, 29]. Affected patients have been shown to have high levels of VEGF and significantly lower levels of IL-35 [30, 31].

The inflammatory cascade and synovial neoangiogenesis drive specific structural changes related to RA pathology. Synovial hypertrophy is related to abnormal proliferation of dysfunctional fibroblast-like synoviocytes (FLS), resistant to apoptosis. FLS sustain joint damage by the secretion of MMPs and tissue inhibitors of metalloproteinases. Cartilage damage is induced by the action of MMPs which cause disassembly of the type II collagen network. Also, chondrocyte apoptosis is enhanced by cytokine, mainly IL-1 and IL-17A. Inflammatory cytokines promote bone erosion through pro-osteoclastogenic effects. Also, osteoclast differentiation may be induced via immune complexes and antigen-binding of ACPA on osteoclast precursors. Bone erosions are usually located at the site where the joint capsule inserts on the periosteum [32, 33].

3. Rheumatoid arthritis: clinical aspects

3.1 Clinical picture of early arthritis

One of the most important things to remember about RA is that it should be diagnosed as early as possible. This is of paramount importance since rheumatoid arthritis is a disease characterized by structural bone lesions that lead to bone deformity and functional disability. However, trying to make an early diagnosis of this disease can prove to be extremely difficult sometimes, and that is because there is no specific or particular symptom or sign of either early or very early RA (eRA).

Moreover, the 2010 European League Against Rheumatism/American College of Rheumatology (EULAR/ACR) classification criteria for RA, which tries to capture patients as early as possible, is to be applied ONLY to people having at least one joint with CLINICAL SYNOVITIS [34]. But, even when synovitis is present, it is not always the expression of early RA.

While early signs and symptoms of RA can be mimicked by other diseases, there are some which should be taken into consideration, such as fatigue, minimal joint pain, joint warmth, joint stiffness, limping, reduction of range of motion, fever, anemia, and depression. It is easy to see that all these are not at all specific, not even for full blown rheumatoid arthritis and even less so for early/very eRA [35].

The interest of knowing how to interpret symptoms in eRA derives from multiple reasons, one of the most important being that it would be extremely useful (on a personal, as well as a societal level) to be able to predict, based on the symptoms of people, who will develop RA and who will not. Unfortunately, with the knowledge we have today, this is not yet feasible. There are still too few studies designed especially for assessing symptoms during this initial period of the disease [36].

Nevertheless, if one tries to group the symptoms which may appear during the early stages of RA, one can delineate three categories [37]:

a. Non-specific symptoms: which are in fact, general (systemic) symptoms produced through the intervention of pro-inflammatory cytokines, which may, thus, intervene in any inflammatory disease, articular or not. Among them, we can outline fatigue, a general feeling of being "un-wellbeing," anxiety, depression, non-specific myalgia or sharp/dull pain near the joints but not in the joints. Sometimes there is low-grade unexplained fever and, rather frequently, sleep disturbances which worsen the general feeling of being "un-wellbeing." To take just one example, fatigue, which is a very common and, frequently, overlooked symptom in RA, correlates with active disease in the sense that it is more pronounced when the disease activity is higher. Its origin is not well understood; it may be the response of the organism to the presence of chronic inflammation, mediated by the action of IL-6. Poor sleep and anemia can contribute to fatigue in RA. This symptom can affect relationships, emotions, mood, productivity, creativity, the general feeling of happiness. Fatigue from RA can associate with poor appetite and weight loss [35].

All these non-specific symptoms may appear in variable proportions in people affected by eRA and their importance resides in the significance pertaining to the risk of a person presenting these symptoms, to develop established RA.

b. Symptoms related to the joints; may vary from mild joint stiffness (sometimes, without having the so-called characteristics of inflammatory joint stiffness) to non-explicable, non-specific joint pain, usually of short duration, with no local signs of inflammation of the joint. As one can see, these are also totally unspecific to the possibility of later developing RA; which is why their presence should prompt a very careful evaluation. On the other hand, when people complain of joint pain, diagnosing them might be easier as pain can motivate people to see a doctor.

c. Symptoms related to functional capacity. These symptoms interfere with one's ability to perform daily living activities. For instance, when one is not capable of performing the opposing movement of the thumb, and hence, not able to make a fist, one will not be able to open a jar's lid. Likewise, if the symptoms are located in the lower limbs, one might not be able to walk or wear shoes. As can be ascertained, these are elements of functional disability that one can encounter in the established RA patient, as well as in other diseases. Therefore, as these are also non-specific to the early phase of RA, they should also be evaluated with care, to reach a correct diagnosis, more so a therapeutic one.

Regardless of the category of symptoms an individual has, the interpretation of their significance is much more difficult and doctors would like to be able to have some hints as to WHAT should he investigate in order not to miss the right diagnosis, in the given window of opportunity. Investigations should be primarily directed to populations or subjects at high risk including female gender, smoking, alcohol, obesity, unhealthy dietary intake, having a family member diagnosed with RA, presence of ACPA, poor dental health, low socioeconomic status. As such, people having symptoms of the above and also one or more of the mentioned risk factors should be given the most attention in assessing their presenting health condition [38].

One other method used to evaluate symptoms of eRA is to, retrospectively, question patients with established RA about their original symptoms [39], followed by making appropriate questionnaires, which are to be used prospectively, to make an early diagnosis. Such an analysis of the literature on this topic was made by Stack et al. and, reviewing 26 papers concentrating on the way patients diagnosed with RA reported their initial symptoms, they found 5 "themes" that describe patient's initial complaints [39].

The first is concerning the swelling of the joint. It was often described as being severe and was most frequently localized at the hands and feet [40–42]. It also has an impact on the ability to perform activities of daily living [43, 44]. Patients reported that it was a progressive feature [45, 46] and that it was sometimes associated with some degree of joint pain [47, 48]. These findings suggest that it might be rational to closely monitor a person complaining of recent onset sensation of joint swelling, even if the swelling itself is not apparent to the doctor.

The second theme used by established RA patients to retrospectively describe their initial symptoms is one of pain and local sensibility, with multiple localizations, again, more frequently, on the hands and feet [49–52] and rarely on the shoulders and hips. Two rather descriptive patterns were identified:

a. gradual occurrence of pain: the most often used descriptors were "episodic pain," "gradual pain," "easy pain," "vague pain." The interpretation given by patients was usually taking into account the activities performed during the day, therefore not much attention was given to the pain until it became persistent and higher in intensity [53–55];

b. acute onset of pain: the most often used descriptors in this circumstance, were "severe pain," "resistant pain," "disability provoking pain," "unbearable pain." Some of the patients describe the occurrence of pain like an "on-off switch" phenomenon. Most often, this pattern was rapidly followed by the occurrence of other symptoms, as well. As such, this kind of joint pain is the one that will get the patient to visit the doctor much faster [45, 46, 55].

The third theme of patients' symptoms is joint stiffness. Quite surprisingly, this was very briefly mentioned and patients never gave a full description, neither was any emphasis put on the significance of the term [46]. In some instances, it was associated with other symptoms, such as fatigue and swelling of the joint [55].

The fourth theme reported retrospectively by patients with established RA, to describe their initial symptoms, is fatigue and muscular weakness [56]. Some patients have reported this as the impossibility to "lift my food tray" [57] or to "lift my toddler" [43]. It appears that fatigue is a really important feature of the beginning of eRA [56]. Some patients even described a "flu-like" sensation of muscular weakness all over their bodies [58].

The fifth and last theme that patients referred to when remembering their initial symptoms of RA is the emotional impact of prolonged suffering [55, 59–61]. It is easily conceivable that a state of sustained discomfort in which the patient does not know for how long it will last and how it may evolve will produce emotional distress. Due to this, patients reported feelings of fear, anger, anxiety, uncertainty, ambivalence. For some patients, this emotional impact was so strong that they had depression and even suicidal ideation [59]. When the emotional disturbance is significant, finding a diagnosis, even that of established RA, comes as a relief [60].

These five themes revealed by Stack et al. are useful for daily clinical practice due to the fact that they can point out of the mass of patients that a physician sees every day, those that the physician should actively follow closely, in order to be able to make the right diagnosis of (preferably) eRA, if this should be the case [39].

Since RA is a systemic disease, potentially affecting any organ system in the body, in the proper context, some of the extraarticular manifestations of the disease, can point out the necessity to further search for a correct diagnosis. Of the numerous such manifestations, one should perhaps remember the following, as a possible manifestation of eRA: peripheral nerve entrapment (e.g. carpal tunnel syndrome), "idiopathic" pulmonary fibrosis or nodules, unexplained amyloidosis, cardiac nodules of unknown origin, cutaneous nodules (that can and should probably be biopsied when unexplained), "idiopathic" vasculitis [38].

As we know, in 2014, Zhao et al. developed classification criteria for eRA, which take into account both clinical and biological aspects of the disease and perform at a variable but acceptable specificity and sensitivity [62, 63]. Nevertheless, they imply that the presence of clinically evident arthritis; and this is, sometimes, not eRA, since everybody tries to make the diagnosis as early as possible! Therefore, these criteria are useful but will miss some of the early or very early RA cases.

One must not forget that we also have the EULAR recommendations on treatment of eRA [64], which state, as one of the overarching principles that "A definitive diagnosis in a patient with early arthritis should only be made after a careful history taking and clinical examination, which should also guide laboratory testing and additional procedures," while in the recommendations it is mentioned that "Clinical examination is the method of choice for detecting arthritis" and that "if a definite diagnosis cannot be reached and the patient has early undifferentiated arthritis, risk factors for persistent and/or erosive disease, including number of swollen joints, acute phase reactants, rheumatoid factor, ACPA and imaging findings, should be considered in management decisions. Patients at risk of persistent arthritis should be started on DMARDs as early as possible (ideally, within 3 months), even if they do not fulfill classification criteria for an inflammatory rheumatological disease." Thus, EULAR provides us with some guidance as to how to attempt to make a diagnosis as early as possible, as well as following it swiftly with the correct management [64].

Identifying (especially) seronegative future established RA patients in the earliest stage of their disease is a difficult endeavor. Until now, we do not know for certain if the symptoms of a person are, by themselves, enough to efficiently stratify the risk of a person to develop established RA [65]. And this is an important unmet need in the field of RA, which precludes continuous study to lower the pressure on the healthcare system, by preventing the major, often irreversible, disabilities associated with this disease, through better early diagnostic expertise.

3.2 Established rheumatoid arthritis

Joint pain is the universal characteristic in RA patients, but the long-standing disease has several features, easily recognizable by a trained rheumatologist, but often misdiagnosed by other specialists. The key to the recognition of the clinical and physical findings of RA is the capability to recognize the outcome of the synovial proliferation and inflammation [66]. As was already stated before, RA can affect any peripheral joints, with predilection on the small joints of the hands and feet, followed by the elbow, shoulder, ankle or knee.

3.2.1 Hand and wrist

Hand and wrist involvement with secondary deformity is a typical feature of late RA [67, 68]. If in the eRA, the physical findings are not extensive, in the late disease one can identify an entire panel of changes. The late, irreversible and most prevalent changes in hands include "swan-neck" and "boutonnière" deformities, along with metacarpophalangeal joints (MCP) swelling, subluxation and "ulnar drift," or ulnar deviation (**Figure 1**). Swelling of the MCP and wrists joints, together with atrophy of the intrinsic muscles of the hand, leads to the aspect of the hand like "two-humped camel's back," while the ulnar deviation makes it similar to the "mole's paw." Persistent inflammation adjacent to ulnar styloid, together with the laxity of the radioulnar ligament leads to a movement of the styloid under the examiner's pressure, similar to the "piano key" [68].

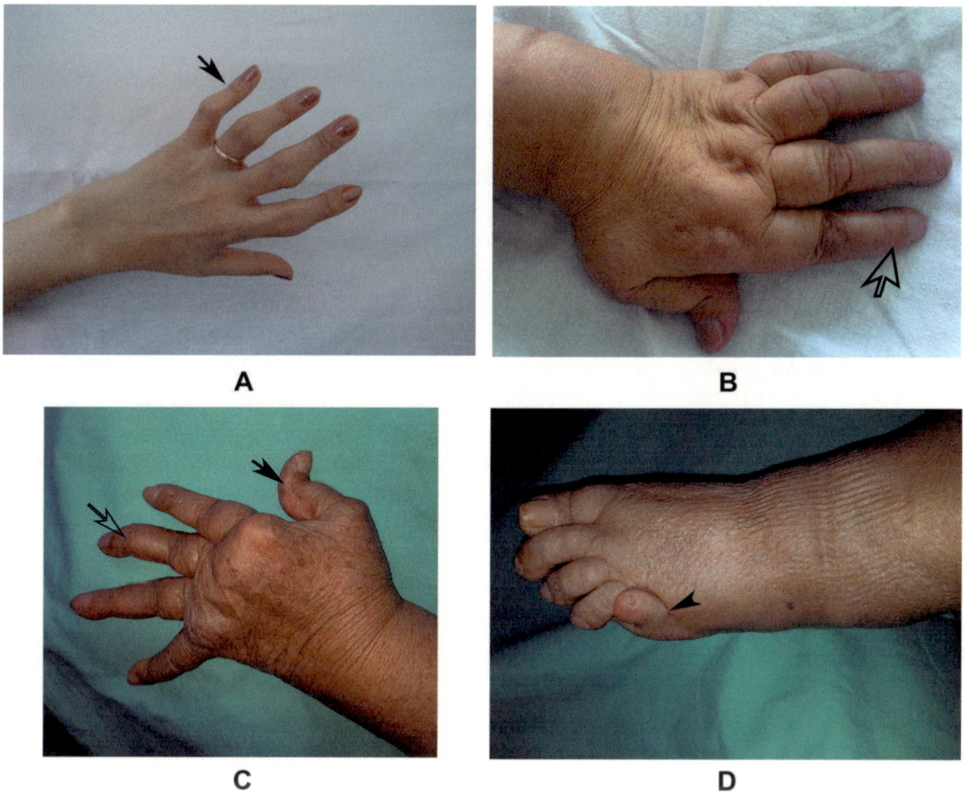

Figure 1.
Images of the small joints of the hands and feet, showing boutonnière - arrow (A and C), swan-neck – Empty arrow (B and C) and hammer toes deformities – arrowhead (D).

The boutonnière deformity presumes the flexion of the proximal interphalangeal (PIP) joint and extension of the distal interphalangeal (DIP) joint [69], whereas the swan-neck, by contrast, means hyperextension of the PIP and flexion of the DIP [68, 70]. The cause of the boutonnière deformity is the lesion of the central slip of the extensor tendon, secondary to tenosynovitis and PIP swelling, with the lateral and volar displacement and conversion of the lateral bands of the extensor tendon, into flexors of the PIP joint. In time, shortening of the tendon leads to hyperextension of the DIP joints. If the DIP swelling is disrupting the extensor tendons, the joints will be forced to remain flexed (due to the action of the only remaining tendons, the flexors). Besides, if the bulging of the PIP is volar, the lateral bands subluxate dorsally, generating hyperextension in the PIP joint and the aspect of the swan-neck deformity.

The involvement of the thumb results in severe functional impairment, due to the loss of the grip between the index finger and the tip of the thumb. The most prevalent pathological aspect of the thumb in RA is one of a “flails,” followed by the boutonnière deformity, which is the same as described before, just one joint back proximally [66].

Extensor tenosynovitis might lead to tendon ruptures, especially at the level of the 6th compartment of extensors, while flexor tendon involvement includes besides thickening of the tendon sheet that could generate either “trigger finger” or a carpal tunnel syndrome [66].

It is not uncommon that the same hand develops different deformities simultaneously leading to a major impact on hand function and subsequently on the ability to perform daily life activities [70].

3.2.2 The elbow

The elbow is often involved both early and in longstanding rheumatoid arthritis. Because of its unique role in maneuvering and positioning the hand in space, the loss of normal motion and stability, or increased pain with the use of this joint are all significant sources of impairment in patients with RA [71]. Synovitis of the elbow joint can be identified by palpation between the olecranon and the epicondyles, especially the lateral one. Olecranon bursitis is a common finding in patients with RA but should be differentiated from the one appearing in polyarticular gout. To mention, in RA it tends to be more frequently bilateral [66].

3.2.3 The shoulder involvement

The shoulder joint is a complex joint and because of its deep location it is difficult to confirm accurately the joint effusion, or the rotator cuff tears only by physical examination, therefore shoulder lesions are often under diagnosed [72]. When involved, it might generate limitation of motion in all planes, with suggestive secondary scapulothoracic movement, or "shoulder pad" sign. The pain generated by joint effusion, subacromial subdeltoid bursitis, or rotator cuff tendon tears is often referred into the deltoid muscle. The fluid inside the biceps tendon sheet is not uncommon [72].

3.2.4 The knee joints

Knee joint synovitis is a frequent finding in patients with RA, anterior swelling being easily detectable through clinical examination, by the "bulge sign" or the ballottement of the patella with the index finger downwards, into the fluid. The Baker cyst is a benign fluctuant swelling of the gastrocnemius-semimembranosus bursa in the popliteal fossa at the back of the knee [73], resulted after severe effusion at the level of the knee joint. Hip joint involvement is associated with pain over the greater trochanter, probably due to bursitis and pain elicited by Patrick's test, or Flexion-Abduction-External Rotation maneuver (FABER) [74].

3.2.5 The ankle involvement

The ankle is an important weight-bearing joint, with a lot of structures involved in RA. Synovitis is common at the level of the tibiotalar subtalar and talonavicular joints, with a high impact on the patient's quality of life [75]. Tenosynovitis of the medial or lateral compartments is increasing the functional impairment. The forefoot comes with specific changes, including calluses under the metatarsal heads and secondary ulcerations, or joint deformities leading to the "hammertoes" aspect (**Figure 1**), resembling the piano hammer [66].

3.2.6 Other types of involvement

Bilateral pain, tenderness, swelling and limitation of jaw movements might be the result of temporomandibular joint involvement and due to these symptoms, patients experience limitations in their daily activities, such as eating, speaking and swallowing.

The involvement of the cervical spine is the most serious skeletal manifestation in patients with RA. Instabilities of the upper cervical spine can lead to headache, neck pain, paresthesias, weakness, signs of vertebrobasilar insufficiency or neurological complications such as bowel and bladder sphincter impairment [66].

3.2.7 Extraarticular features of RA

Most frequent extraarticular features of RA are represented by the *rheumatoid nodules*, with subcutaneous disposition on the extensor surfaces and joints at sites of chronic mechanical irritation and typical clinical characteristics [76, 77]. The diagnosis requires sometimes biopsy to differentiate them from gouty tophi but need no specific treatment unless they are causing pain, interference in mechanical function, nerve compression, or other important local phenomena. It is uncommon to find nodules within the first year from the disease onset, whereas it is more like a longstanding disease feature. To note, that patients with rheumatoid nodules are at an increased risk of developing other severe extraarticular manifestation. Association of HLA-DRB1*04 gene and smoking were found to be important predictors for the extraarticular disease [77].

Hematological abnormalities are not uncommon, especially anemia of different causes, such as chronic inflammatory disease, through hepcidin intervention and blockage of iron inside macrophages, or secondary to the gastrointestinal complication of the anti-inflammatory treatment or loss of folic acid during methotrexate therapy. Thrombocytopenia is uncommon, usually drug-induced. More frequently, RA patients manifest thrombocytosis of unknown cause, but correlated with disease activity and involved joint count. Lymphadenopathy is frequent in active RA, with a benign histological pattern, usually located in axillary, inguinal or epitrochlear areas. The lymph nodes are usually not painful and mobile [76].

Felty's syndrome represents the association of RA with splenomegaly and leukopenia (neutropenia) and usually occurs in seropositive patients with longstanding, deforming disease with rheumatoid nodules present. Some of those patients may also present thrombocytopenia and extremity ulcerations (lower leg) and hyperpigmentation of the skin, and are positive for antinuclear antibodies. To mention an increased risk of opportunistic infections, due to neutropenia [78].

Hepatic involvement is non-specific and minimal, related mostly to treat adverse effects, with an increase of liver enzymes that should decrease with discontinuation of the incriminated drug. On the other hand, in up to 65% of patients with Felty's syndrome, there are liver abnormalities, from portal fibrosis and abnormal lobular architecture to nodular regenerative hyperplasia [77, 78].

Pulmonary complications of RA are frequent, with men being more often affected than women and include pleural disease, in up to 50% in autopsies studies, parenchymal peripheral pulmonary asymptomatic nodules (PPP nodules), that can measure up to 8 cm in diameter, diffuse interstitial pulmonary fibrosis, or bronchiolitis obliterans organizing pneumonia (BOOP). Pulmonary nodules and pneumoconiosis appear in patients with RA and extensive exposure to coal dust (Caplan's syndrome), silica and asbestos. The RA- associated interstitial pneumonitis should be distinguished from the one generated by the methotrexate toxicity, the last one usually having a subacute onset, with low radiographic evidence of fibrosis, but rapid symptom progression. Inflammation of the cricoarytenoid joint might lead to other respiratory complications – upper airways obstruction [76, 79].

Heart disease presumes all cardiac structures involvement by intricate complex mechanisms of nodule formation, vasculitis of the coronary arteries, amyloidosis, serositis, valvulitis or fibrosis. Pericarditis is the most common cardiac feature of heart involvement, usually asymptomatic [80, 81]. Myocardial disease secondary to granulomatous lesions similar to rheumatoid nodules can lead to arrhythmia. Valvular granulomatous lesions might generate dysfunctionalities at the level of the mitral and aortic valves.

Rheumatoid vasculitis is a panarteritis, with mononuclear cells infiltrate and fibrinoid necrosis, which leads to clinical manifestations such as peripheral neuropathy, palpable purpura or visceral infarcts. It is frequently associated with increased RF, erosive disease and rheumatoid nodules [80].

Other extraarticular manifestations of RA include *neurological impairment*, secondary to mononeuritis multiplex, to nerve compression by synovial proliferation (carpal tunnel syndrome) or to atlantoaxial subluxation; *eye involvement* includes keratoconjunctivitis sicca, episcleritis or scleromalacia perforans (secondary to a perforating rheumatoid nodule). Glucocorticoids might cause glaucoma and cataracts and chloroquine derivates cause retinopathy; the gastrointestinal disease can be secondary to mesenteric or hepatic vasculitis or associated with anti-inflammatory treatment [77].

Amyloidosis might complicate RA in up to 0.7% of patients with longstanding disease, leading to a poor outcome, with only 58% survival rates at 4 years [76].

Bone involvement is also frequent in rheumatoid arthritis patients, secondary to osteoclastic hyperactivity and or osteoblastic hypoactivity, in patients with impaired moving, local effect of proinflammatory cytokines or to the adverse effect of glucocorticoids [82].

Muscle atrophy is frequent, especially near affected joints. Inflammatory myositis or glucocorticoid myopathy (usually with the use of higher doses) might be present in patients with RA [76, 77].

4. Rheumatoid arthritis: imaging

Recent advances in the imaging field and therapeutic possibilities are changing the outcome in RA. Still, conventional radiology (CR) represents the main imaging method for rheumatoid arthritis patients' evaluation, in daily practice. The treat to target approach has brought into attention the new methods, ultrasonography (US) and magnetic resonance imaging (MRI), as more sensitive and specific imaging modalities. In this way, CR remains a method for identifying old and late changes, lesions that already happened, while US and MRI are the methods for identifying acute inflammatory lesions and details of small structural changes. Other methods, such as arthrography, computer tomography (CT) or scintigraphy remain suitable for complex cases and will not be subject to our paper [77].

Conventional radiology, a cheap and widely available method shows a wide spectrum of changes at the level of the peripheral joints, including hands, wrists, feet, and ankles or even larger joints (knee, shoulder, elbow), depending on the disease duration. Thus, imaging of any joint disorder, including rheumatoid arthritis should start with this method [77].

Peripheral joint involvement shows typical radiographic changes in rheumatoid arthritis including soft tissue swelling related to joint effusion or synovitis, juxta-articular osteoporosis, joint space narrowing and the late disease changes, bone erosions, and ankylosis. To note, the fact that joint space narrowing (JSN) is a good indicator for hyaline cartilage loss, as the articular space is mainly composed of the two-cartilage thickness sum, normally about 2 mm [83]. A comparison with adjacent or contralateral joints might clarify narrowing. Erosions occur earliest at the level of the carpal bones, especially pisiform or triquetrum, at the level of the ulnar styloid and second metacarpophalangeal (MCP) joint, in the bare area (metacarpal head, with no cartilage) [84]. Studies showed that up to 30% of the patients do not develop erosions in the first 2 years from disease onset, but still, most of the patients do, a fact that led to the expert recommendation of repeating CR every 6–12 months in eRA and every 1–2 years in late disease [85].

To quantify lesions and for a better follow-up of the disease, Sharp proposed a scoring system of erosions and JSN of hands [86]. The modified Sharp score, proposed by Van der Heijde, included feet, for a total of 16 areas evaluated for erosions and 15 for

JSN in each hand and 6 areas for erosions and six for JSN in each foot [87]. Radiographic progression can redefine remission, as clinically quiet joints often progress.

CR of the spine might show some abnormalities, especially in the cervical segment, which is involved in more than half of the patient [85]. The most frequent finding in this area is atlantoaxial subluxation and basilar invagination [88, 89], both identified best in a lateral radiograph, with the flexed neck. For the diagnosis of atlantoaxial subluxation, one should measure the distance between the anterior arch of C1 and anterior aspect of the dens of C2. Expected values in normal subjects should not exceed 3 mm in adults and 5 mm in children. The distance higher than those cutoffs lead to a diagnosis of subluxation and the ones higher than 8 mm require surgical intervention. Basilar invagination diagnosis should be confirmed by MRI or CT [88].

US was recently included by EULAR recommendations on the use of imaging, between the techniques with a potential role in RA diagnosis and management [90, 91]. The reflection of ultrasound waves by body structures generates US images of those structures in the greyscale (GS) [92]. Adding the Doppler technique to the examination, we obtain information on the blood flow inside structures. The higher the ultrasound frequency, the higher the detail on the image, but lower penetrance. In reverse, the lower the frequency, the higher penetrance, but with a low-quality image. Therefore, the use of appropriate probe frequencies is required for an optimal US evaluation. The higher frequency transducers (e.g. 10–18 MHz) are mandatory for superficial structures, such as small joints of the hands and feet and ligaments and tendons, whereas lower frequency probes (e.g. 5–12 MHz) are useful for deeper joints, such as hip, knee or shoulder [90].

For most of the joints, US allows visualization of most features of rheumatoid arthritis, including joint effusion, synovial hypertrophy, bursitis, tenosynovitis or bone erosions, being more sensitive than clinical examination for depicting subclinical synovitis and other inflammatory (**Figure 2**), acute changes and more sensitive than CR for detection of bony structural changes, like erosions [93, 94].

The outcome measurement in the rheumatology group (OMERACT), under the EULAR umbrella, developed definitions for all the US findings in rheumatology, which should be confirmed in two perpendicular planes. Thus, effusion is defined as abnormal hypoechoic or anechoic intraarticular material, that can be displaced and compressed, with no Doppler signal, whereas synovial hypertrophy or proliferation is defined as abnormal hypoechoic intraarticular tissue that is not displaceable and compressible but may exhibit Doppler signal [95].

Other inflammatory, acute, feature of RA is tenosynovitis, identified by the US as hypoechoic or anechoic thickened tissue with or without fluid within the tendon sheath, which is seen in two perpendicular planes and which may exhibit Doppler signal (**Figure 3**) [95].

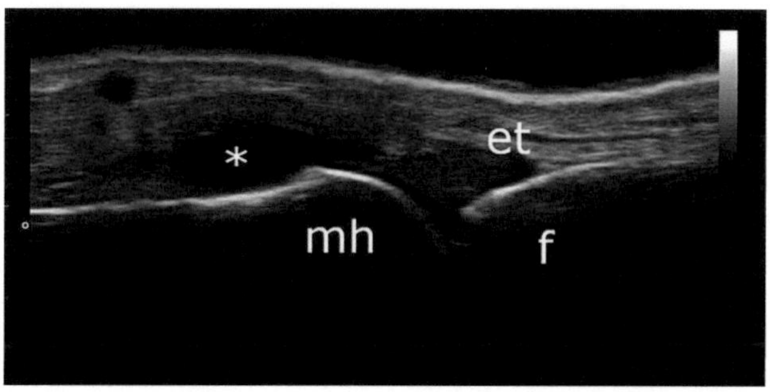

Figure 2.
US images showing - synovitis of MCP joint (asterisk – synovitis, mh – metacarpal head, f – phalanx, et – extensor tendon). Original image, from the personal archive (FLORIN VREJU).

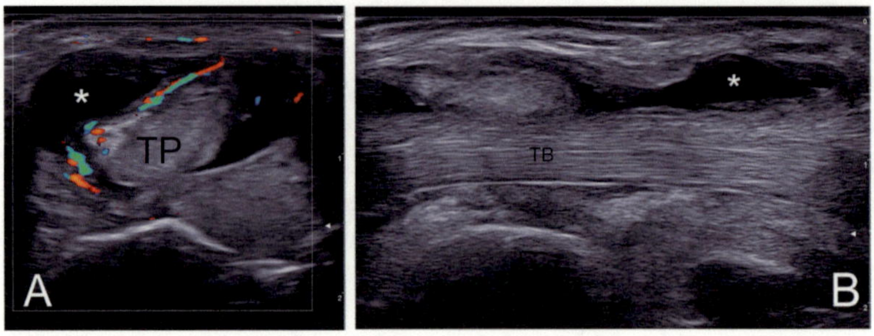

Figure 3.
US images showing - tenosynovitis of the tibialis posterior (asterisk – tenosynovitis) in transverse, with Doppler activity (A) and longitudinal scan (B).

4.1 Original image, from personal archive (FLORIN VREJU)

Since the US is more and more used in daily practice both for diagnosis and monitoring disease, a scoring system for synovitis became mandatory. The most used is the one proposed by Szkudlarek et al. [96] that scored fluid as follows: grade 0 – no effusion, grade 1 – minimal amount of fluid, grade 2 – moderate (no distension of the joint capsule) and grade 3 – extensive fluid collection (with distension of the joint capsule). The synovial hypertrophy was scored as grade 0 – none, grade 1 – minimal synovial thickening, grade 2 – synovial thickening bulging over the line linking top of bone cortical (no extension along bone diaphysis), grade 3 – synovial thickening bulging over the line, with extension to at list one of the bone diaphysis. Semiquantitative grading included grade 0 – no flow, grade 1 – single vessel signal, grade 2 – Doppler signal in less than half of the area of synovium and grade 3 – Doppler signal over more than half of the synovial area (**Figure 4**). Recently was developed a new combined score, Global OMERACT – EULAR Sonography Scoring (GLOESS), which considered the higher score of GS or power Doppler (PD) as the score for the joint [97].

The most characteristic US finding in RA is bone erosion, defined as an intraarticular step-down discontinuity of the bone surface that is visible in two perpendicular planes [95]. Scoring system for erosions according to Szkudlarek et al. defined grade 0 as normal bone cortical, grade 1 as bone irregularities, but without defect in two perpendicular planes, grade 2 – the defect is seen in two perpendicular planes, grade 3 – extensive bone destruction [96]. A more accurate grading score for erosions was the one based on irregularity size: grade 0 – no erosions, grade 1 – erosion <1 mm, grade 2 – small erosion between 1 and 1.9 mm, grade 3 – moderate erosion, between 2 and 4 mm, grade 4 – dimensions higher than 4 mm [98].

Validity of the method and sensitivity to change were primarily demonstrated for all US findings by Terslev et al. [99, 100], thus making it an important imaging method in the management of RA, along with other studies which confirmed predicting value in the treatment response [101, 102], and the role in discriminating between clinical and imaging, real remission [93, 103, 104].

However, even if the diagnosis is enhanced and not made only by the US and even if it is highly operator dependent, ultrasonography offers a cheap and dynamic possibility for monitoring the disease activity and progression and for assessing the persistence of subclinical inflammation in RA [92, 93].

Magnetic resonance imaging represents a favored and favorite imaging method in inflammatory joint diseases, as it allows evaluation of all the structures involved in those pathologies, being able to depict synovitis, tenosynovitis, erosions and more than this, the bone marrow edema, a feature that remains hidden to the

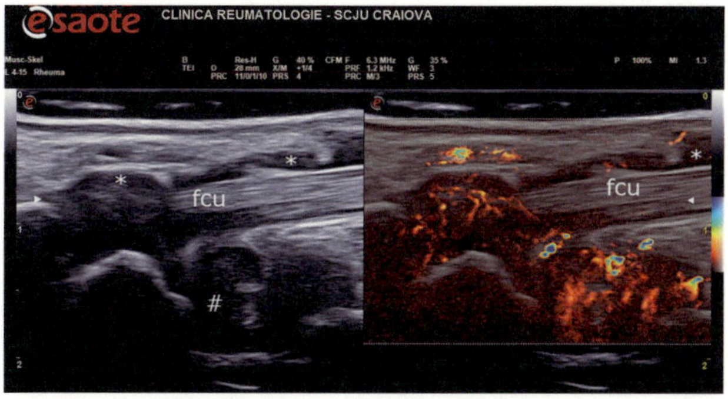

Figure 4.
US images showing - tenosynovitis of flexor carpi ulnaris and wrist synovitis, with Doppler signal present (asterisk – tenosynovitis, fcu – flexor carpi ulnaris, # – wrist synovitis).

US. MRI sequences that can be useful in RA patients include T1-weighted (T1w), favored by short imaging times and good anatomical details, T2-weighted (T2w) and short tau inversion recovery (STIR), both good for depicting inflammation, such as bone marrow edema or synovitis [105]. Adding intravenous contrast agent, like paramagnetic gadolinium (Gd) to T1w sequences allows us to visualize detailed structural lesions and, at the same time, the tissue vascularity and perfusion, inflamed synovium being easily recognizable. It is always advisable to use two sequences in parallel, to compare high signals in the water-sensitive (WS) one (T2w or STIR) with high-resolution details in the fat sensitive one (T1w). Thus, one can identify active erosions, by a hyperintense signal in WS sequences and hypointense signals in the T1w image [105].

As a conclusion, MRI allows identification of synovitis, tenosynovitis, and erosions and proves to be an important tool in the diagnosis, in the disease activity monitoring and treatment response. However, even if it brings complete information on the peripheral joints, the use of MRI in RA patients in clinical practice remains lower in comparison to US and CR, due to issues related to availability, cost, and duration of an examination. More than this, it cannot offer a dynamic assessment of structures [77].

5. Rheumatoid arthritis: pharmacotherapy

According to guidelines, the therapeutic approach for RA patients includes an early start of conventional synthetic disease-modifying antirheumatic drugs (csDMARDs), followed by biologic DMARDs (bDMARDs) and targeted synthetic DMARDs, aimed at a low disease activity or remission.

Regarding csDMARDs, Methotrexate (MTX) remains the first therapeutic choice, due to its immunomodulatory and immunosuppressive action, efficacy and sustained effect; it is administered orally or subcutaneous, with doses starting from 7.5–10 mg weekly up to 20–25 mg/week, In case of MTX intolerance, leflunomide (10/20 mg/day) or sulfasalazine (2–3 g/day) should be considered as therapeutic agents [106]. Treatment monitoring requires CBC, ALT, AST and creatinine evaluation at baseline, every 2–4 weeks for the first 3 months, every 8–12 weeks for the next 3–6 months and every 12 weeks after. Screening for hepatitis B and C should be performed before initiating the treatment. An increase over three times of hepatic enzymes requires treatment interruption [106].

If the therapeutic target is not achieved with csDMARD therapy, bDMARDs or tsDMARDs should represent the next approach (**Figure 5**) [106].

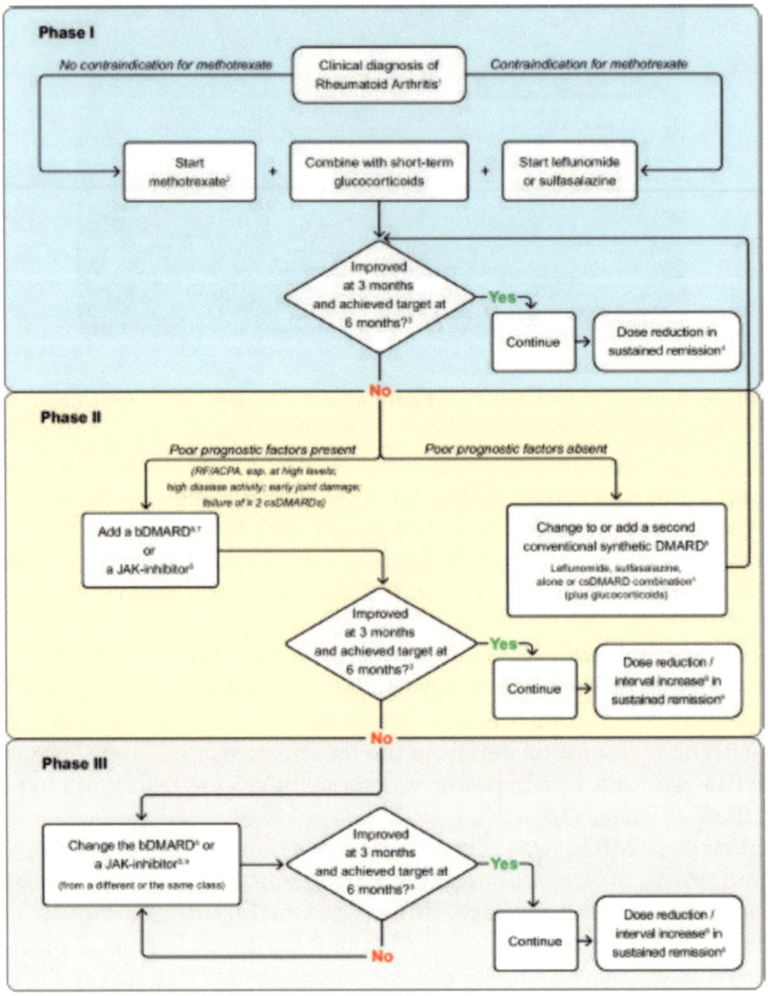

Figure 5.
EULAR recommendations for the management of rheumatoid arthritis with synthetic and biological disease-modifying antirheumatic drugs [106].

5.1 Biologic agents

Rheumatoid inflammation is initiated and maintained through immunological pathways when activated T and B cells produce cytotoxins – directly toxic to tissues – and cytokines such as TNF and interleukins (IL-1 and IL-6) – which provide further amplifies the interaction between pro-inflammatory cells [107, 108]. Biologic bDMARDs are licensed for the treatment of moderate-to-severe RA and target specific T and B-cell activation by [107, 109]:

1. Inhibiting TNF (with excessive production in the synovial fluid in RA) and reducing the progression of joint damage:

   - Adalimumab,

   - Certolizumab,

   - Etanercept,

- Golimumab,
- Infliximab

2. Binding of the CD80/86 receptor and preventing co-stimulation interaction between T cells:

- Abatacept

3. Blocking the IL-1 receptor:

- Anakinra

4. Blocking the IL-6 receptor and presenting a better safety profile:

- Tocilizumab

5. Producing B-cell depletion and reducing the accumulation of bone damaging oxygen-free radicals:

- Rituximab

Early use of bDMARDs can improve patient outcomes, reduce the symptoms of RA and modify the course of the disease, leading to remissions that can last several years [110].

Biosimilars are highly similar molecules with equivalent therapeutic effect to bDMARDs, also prescribed in RA, to reduce treatment costs because they are authorized by comparing randomized controlled trial data [109]. Biologic agents may be effective when DMARDs therapy fails to bring improvement of the physical function, but they present higher costs due to their complex manufacturing process [107, 109]. Biologic agents are genetically derived from living human or animal cells as whole monoclonal antibodies or as a specific fragment of an antibody called fusion protein [109].

Therefore, their protein structure predisposes patients to increased risk for infection, reactivation of latent tuberculosis, development of lupus-type reaction (mostly characterized by rashes, leukopenia, and thrombocytopenia) and vasculitis [107, 109, 111].

Pre-existing airway disease and interstitial lung disease have shown worsening symptoms and increased mortality after administering biological RA treatment [111].

Therapy monitoring: all patients should perform tuberculin skin testing or interferon-gamma release assay (IGRA) blood test before commencing anti-rheumatic treatment with biologic agents. Pre-existing airway disease and interstitial lung disease have shown worsening symptoms and increased mortality after administering biological RA treatment [110]. Neurological complications similar to multiple sclerosis symptoms and demyelinating disorders have also been associated with bDMARDs treatment and regular monitoring for new skin cancer is necessary regarding all patients receiving biologic agents [111]. Patients should not receive live vaccines during treatment, except for pneumococcal, influenza and hepatitis B which are killed vaccines [107, 109, 112]. Neurological complications similar to multiple sclerosis symptoms and demyelinating disorders have also been associated with bDMARDs treatment and regular monitoring for new skin cancer is necessary regarding all patients receiving biologic agents.

The bDMARDs have different pharmacokinetics properties and dosage, but similar adverse reactions and contraindications for the TNF inhibitors (TNFi). All TNFi increases cardiac mortality in RA patients with associated congestive heart failure (class III/IV and an ejection fraction of 50% or less) [107, 109]. Lymphoproliferative cancers, especially in children and adolescents, have been reported after using

TNFi, therefore the US Food and Drug Administration (FDA) added a black box warning product labeling. Patients are recommended to use appropriate skin protection. TNFi does not increase the risk of congenital malformation and is classified as pregnancy category B (no documented human toxicity) [110, 113]. However, due to the intense placental transfer of Ig in the third trimester, TNFi may increase the risk of neonatal bacterial and fungal infections. The lowest risk appears in etanercept and certolizumab, which are preferred for administration [113].

All in all, the following screening tests should be performed before initiating bDMARDs therapy:

1. Full infection history and screen, chest radiographs, tuberculin skin test, IGRA, asses risk factors for HIV, hepatitis B and C screening to exclude the presence of bacterial or viral infection;

2. Full blood count, urinalysis;

3. Check vaccination status;

4. Check the family/patient history of demyelinating disease or malignancy;

5. Review cardiac function;

6. Antibody profile assessment: anti-nuclear antibodies (ANA) and deoxyribonucleic acid (DNA).

5.1.1 Adalimumab

Adalimumab is a TNFi, fully humanized IgG1 monoclonal antibody (MAb), with a lower risk than animal-derived agents of generating immune responses such as injection-site reactions to anaphylaxis. It neutralizes the biological function of TNF, therefore it is recommended in patients with moderate-to-severe active RA, in association with methotrexate (MTX), as 40 mg subcutaneous injection or as monotherapy, with a 40 mg increase dosage once a week if the patient presents low rates of disease response. Pharmacokinetic properties: the average absolute bioavailability following a single 40 mg dose was 64%, with a terminal phase half-life of approximately 2 weeks. Pharmaceutical forms: premixed syringes or injection pens containing 40 mg, which is administered every 14 days. Therapy monitoring and specific screening commune to all bDMARDS: during treatment and 6 months after stopping. Concomitant administration of adalimumab with other bDMARDs (etanercept, anakinra, abatacept) is not recommended based upon the increased risk for infections and other potential pharmacological interactions. FKB327, a biosimilar agent, presented pharmacokinetic equivalence and similar pharmacodynamic properties to adalimumab, with minor differences due to formulation buffers, but not clinically relevant [109, 114, 115]. To highlight their safety of administration in patients with RA, biosimilars are mentioned as highly similar molecules with equivalent therapeutic effect to bDMARDs [109]. Biosimilars are prescribed to reduce treatment costs because they are authorized by comparing randomized controlled trial data [109].

5.1.2 Etanercept

Etanercept is a recombinant human soluble TNF-α receptor, produced in Chinese hamster ovary cells. It was the first TNFi approved by FDA in November 1998 as an immune-suppressant for RA treatment. Other indications for etanercept are: juvenile idiopathic arthritis, spondyloarthritis, and plaque psoriasis. Pharmacokinetic properties: slow absorption and elimination, bioavailability 76%, the long half-life of 70 hours, and the presence of renal or hepatic impairment should not require dosage modification. Dosage: subcutaneous injection, 25 mg twice weekly or 50 mg once weekly. In 2018, its first biosimilar SB-4 also received approval and was developed as a single-use pre-filled syringe available at 25 and 50 mg. SB-4 lacks l-arginine and latex in the needle shield, which may explain the lower risk of injection site reactions in SB-4 treated patients. The most common adverse events are upper respiratory tract infections, nasopharyngitis, and hepatobiliary disorders. Neurological events have rarely been reported [109, 116, 117].

5.1.3 Golimumab

Golimumab, another human MAb, prevents TNF-α binding to its receptors, and it must be administered in combination with MTX in case of failure or intolerance to other TNFi. Pharmacokinetic properties: absolute bioavailability 77%, the terminal half-life of 18 days, passage through placenta and breast milk. Dosage: the starting recommended dosage is 50 mg monthly, by subcutaneous injection, with a visible clinical response after 12–14 weeks of treatment. Treatment should be discontinued if no response appears after administering four doses of 100 mg. Precautions and adverse reactions are similar to other TNFi [107, 109, 118].

5.1.4 Certolizumab

Certolizumab pegol is a recombinant human MAb bound to polyethylene glycol which increases its half-life to approximately 14 days and reduces the risk of antibody-dependent cell-mediated cytotoxicity. It is indicated in associations with MTX for the treatment of moderate-to-severe RA in adult patients, with a recommended starting dose of 400 mg (as 2 subcutaneous injections of 200 mg each in 1 day) at weeks 0, 2 and 4, followed by 200 mg every 2 weeks as a maintenance dosage. Treatment should be discontinued if there is no response after 12 weeks of treatment. Due to its reduced placental transfer, certolizumab is one of the safest biologic agents for use in pregnancy and can be given during all trimesters [107, 109, 113].

5.1.5 Infliximab

Adverse reactions are mostly observed in chimeric biologic agents, such as *infliximab* (which contain only 75% human antibodies), due to the development of neutralizing antibodies also associated with decreased therapeutic effect. Therefore, infliximab, a chimeric human-murine TNFi, which contains combined portions of mouse and human IgG1, must be administered with a low-oral-dose of MTX or prednisone to prevent adverse reactions. Dosage: it is the only monoclonal antibody administered only by intravenous infusion, at a dose of 3 mg/kg at weeks 0, 2 and 6, and maintenance infusions at 8 weeks. A specific and acute infusion reaction presents as fever, pruritus, chills, and rash, after 2 hours of receiving the drug, however, anaphylactic shock rarely appears. Prior 30–60 minutes to infliximab infusion, cetirizine 0.5 mg/kg or hydrocortisone 4 mg/kg and paracetamol 15 mg/kg are necessary to avoid infusion reactions. Lupus-like-syndrome and vasculitis have also been reported. Blood tests should be performed to evaluate the eventual drop of infliximab plasmatic concentration which indicates the appearance of neutralizing antibodies [107–109].

5.1.6 Abatacept

Abatacept is a fusion protein and a non-TNFi biologic medicine, which modulates lymphocyte responses and inflammation by blocking a co-stimulatory signal for T-cell activity. It is always recommended to be used with MTX in highly active RA in patients without positive response in prior treatment with MTX or in patients who have a contraindication preventing them from receiving rituximab, another non-TNFi biologic agent. Pharmacokinetic properties: bioavailability 78%, the terminal half-life of 14 days, placental crossing, but no transfer through breast milk. Dosage: it can be administered as intravenous infusion depending on patient weight: 500 mg <60 kg, 750 mg <100 kg, 1000 mg > 100 kg, every 2 weeks for two initial doses and then every 4 weeks. Abatacept presents better persistence rates over TNFi, even though it is a second line biologic agent [119, 120]. Alternatively, it can be given by the subcutaneous injection of 125 mg once a week. Common adverse reactions include headaches, nasopharyngitis and upper respiratory tract infections, dizziness, back pain, hypertension, dyspepsia, urinary tract infections, rash. Several studies have shown that abatacept is associated with presents a better prognosis than other biologic agents in patients with RA and interstitial lung disease [111]. Precautions should nonetheless be taken in patients older than 65 years, due to the increased number of reported malignancy cases [107, 108].

5.1.7 Rituximab

Rituximab binds to CD20, a protein expressed on B lymphocytes and affects B and T-cell interaction and cytokine production, delaying bone and tissue damage. B-cell recovery takes several months, therefore rituximab has a prolonged effect which allows intermittent therapy based on the reactivation of arthritis symptoms. Dosage: clinical response is usually achieved within 16–24 weeks and both rituximab and its biosimilar are administered in association with MTX for better therapeutic outcomes. The first dose is 1000 mg by intravenous infusion followed by a second dose of 1000 mg after 2 weeks, associated with intravenous methylprednisolone to prevent infusion reactions. The risk of infusion reactions decreases after every administration. Paracetamol and antihistamines may also bring benefits to atopic patients. Rituximab is preferred to be administered to patients with a history of malignancies, due to the fact that rituximab has not been associated with an increased risk of cancer. Contraindications for rituximab refer especially to severe active infections and severe heart failure [107, 109].

5.1.8 Tocilizumab

Tocilizumab binds to membrane receptors specific to IL-6 and therefore inhibits IL-6 which is involved in multiple regulation mechanisms of the immune response, hematopoiesis, and bone metabolism. In RA, IL-6 is responsible for raised platelet count, protein and auto-antibody overproduction, induction of osteoclasts, development of inflammation and joint destruction. Tocilizumab is licensed as a treatment for RA, in association or not with MTX and in patients following other DMARDs failure or intolerance to them. It represents the only therapy that has shown superiority over MTX monotherapy and other DMARDs, although the association with other antirheumatic drugs prolonged retention of tocilizumab [107, 109]. Furthermore, a retrospective observational study in 2019 has shown that tocilizumab and etanercept were the most persistent drugs, referring to retention rate and drug survival, with a median retention duration of 30.9 months. This study demonstrates a higher efficacy specific to tocilizumab [121]. Pharmacokinetic properties: half-life is maintained between 6 and 18 days, depending on concentration and administration rhythm. Due to its mechanism of action, tocilizumab stimulates the action of cytochrome P450, especially CYP1A2, CYP2C9, CYP2C19, and CYP3A4, involved in the metabolism of many other drugs such as statins, warfarin, benzodiazepines, oral contraceptives, calcium channel blockers, theophylline, phenytoin. Tocilizumab increases the need for a higher dosage if associated with these other classes of medicines. Patients receiving tocilizumab will present a reduction in plasmatic neutrophils and platelets, but also a growth in plasmatic lipid levels; treatment should not be initiated in patients with an absolute neutrophil count less than 2×10^9 L and patients should have their cholesterol levels checked 4–8 weeks after initiating treatment with tocilizumab [107, 109, 122]. Further cautions should be taken in patients with aminotransaminase levels greater than 1.5 times the upper limit. Dosage: it can be administered as a subcutaneous injection once a week with a dosage of 162 mg or as an intravenous infusion with a dosage of 8 mg/kg/every 4 weeks, with a maximum of 800 mg per infusion [107, 109, 122].

Supplementary precautions should be taken in pregnancy and administration of rituximab, tocilizumab, and abatacept, due to their limited safety documentation when compared with TNFi [113].

5.1.9 Anakinra

Anakinra is less effective than other biologics, therefore it is not normally recommended, although patients with refractory disease can follow and benefit from this treatment. Failure of treatment in RA patients can be defined as a lack of response in 3 to 6 months after commencing therapy or as a loss of response after a first improvement was registered. Anakinra is a human IL-1 receptor antagonist, given as a subcutaneous injection in combination with weekly MTX. Dosage: 100 mg/per day, administered at approximately the same time each day. Topical glucocorticoids can avoid injectional reactions and are recommended. Specific adverse effects: rashes, urticaria, the elevation of hepatic enzyme levels, reproductive toxicity and a higher risk for serious infections and pulmonary events than other biologic agents, especially when associated with other TNF-antagonists [107, 109, 123].

5.2 Targeted synthetic DMARDs-JAK inhibitors (JAKi)

The multiple cytokines involved in the RA pathogenesis signal through Janus kinase/signal transduction and activator of transcription pathway (JAK-STAT). JAK represents intracellular tyrosine kinases associated with several cytokine receptors. JAK family includes JAK1, JAK2, JAK3, and TYK2 that are paired with specific receptors. Depending on the structure of their receptors, cytokines can be classified in [124]:

1. Type 1 receptors:
    - *γ chain* (IL-2, IL-7, IL-9, IL-15);
    - *gp 130 family* (IL-6, IL-11, oncostatin M-OSM, leukemia inhibitory factor-LIF),
    - *p40 subunit* (IL-12, IL-23)
    - and *β chain cytokines receptors* (IL-3, IL-5, GM-CSF).
2. Type 2 receptors include IL-10 and TNF families.

Recently, RA therapeutic research has focused on intracellular pathways and with advances in technology and disease knowledge, more targeted therapies were developed. JAKi represents an attractive therapeutic resource for patients with active moderate/severe RA, due to their oral bioavailability [124, 125].

Currently, there are two JAKi approved for RA treatment, associated with MTX or as monotherapy: *tofacitinib* (selective for JAK1 and JAK3) and *baricitinib* (selective for JAK1 and JAK2). Also, other agents are undergoing clinical studies: *upadacitinib* and *filgotinib* (selective for JAK1, 74-fold selectivity for the first agent and 28-fold for the second one), *peficitinib* (selective for JAK1 and JAK2) and *decernotinib* (JAK3 selective) [124–127].

5.2.1 Tofacitinib

Tofacitinib, the first oral JAKi approved for RA treatment, is a targeted small synthetic molecule, a reversible competitive inhibitor that binds to ATP binding site of the kinase domain of JAK. It selectively inhibits signaling through cytokine receptors associated with JAK3 and JAK1. Regarding its pharmacologic properties, it has a pharmacokinetic profile directly related to dose, with a half-life of approximately 3 hours. It is metabolized by the liver, via cytochrome P450, primary, and cytochrome P2C19, secondary, and eliminated renal. It is recommended for patients with moderate to severe RA, associated with MTX or in monotherapy, in doses of 5 mg twice a day [126]. Therapy monitoring: complete blood count should be performed at the initiation, 4–8 weeks after and every 3 months afterward. Lipid profile should be evaluated 4–8 weeks after initiation and according to hyperlipidemia guidelines if it is the case. Liver enzymes should be periodically monitored. The recommendations for treatment interruption are presented in **Table 1**.

5.2.2 Baricitinib

As well as *baricitinib*, it should be used carefully in patients with risk factors for deep vein thrombosis (DVT) or pulmonary embolism (PE) (old age, obesity, history of DVT or PE, surgery or immobilization). It is not recommended in case of pregnancy, lactation or children; it is also important to administer with caution in patients over 75 years [127]. Baricitinib, the second agent approved for the treatment

	Monitoring	**Action**
Lipid	4–8/12 weeks after treatment initiation and afterward according to hyperlipidemia guidelines	Management according to hyperlipidemia guidelines
Absolute neutrophil count (ANC)	Before initiation and afterward according to routine patient evaluation	Treatment interruption if ANC is $<1 \times 10^9$cells/L; may be restarted once ANC is above this value
Absolute lymphocyte count (ALC)		Treatment interruption if ANC is $<0.5 \times 10^9$cells/L; may be restarted once ANC is above this value
Hemoglobin (Hb)		Treatment interruption if Hb is <8 g/dL and may be restarted once Hb is above this value
Hepatic aminotransferases		Temporary interruption if drug-induced liver injury is suspected

Table 1.
Monitoring tofacitinib and baricitinib treatment [128].

of RA is a competitive ATP kinase inhibitor, selective inhibitor of JAK1 and JAK2 (100-fold selectivity over JAK3), that reduces immune cell functions by targeting several cytokines (IL-6, IL-12, IL-23, IFNs, and GM-CSF) and growth factor stimulation. By presenting less affinity for JAK3 it may be associated with decreased immunosuppressive effects [128]. After oral administration is very fast absorbed, with a maximum plasmatic concentration of about 90 minutes and a half-life of 14 hours that allows once a day administration. It does not have a significant liver metabolization and is excreted in the urine, mostly unchanged. It is recommended to reduce the dose in case of renal insufficiency, for patients with a creatinine clearance between 30 and 60 mL/minute, and is contraindicated to be administered when the clearance is under 30 mL/minute. It is administered in doses of 4 mg/day. Doses of 2 mg/day should be considered for patients over 75 years, with a history of infections or in case of persistent remission [129]. Safety and side effects: Before therapy initiation, all patients should be tested for latent tuberculosis and viral hepatitis and also baseline analyses must include absolute lymphocyte count (ALC), absolute neutrophil count (ANC) and hemoglobin. Laboratory changes that may be observed are represented by decreased hemoglobin and neutrophils, increased hepatic enzymes, creatinine, low-density, and high-density lipoprotein. Patients monitoring is presented in **Table 1**. During treatment, there were reported cases of tuberculosis reactivation, herpes zoster, malignancy and thrombosis [127].

5.2.3 Upadacitinib

Upadacitinib is an under investigation oral JAKi, with a higher selectivity for JAK1, which provided favorable efficacy, safety, and tolerability in the studies conducted so far. Similar to tofacitinib and baricitinib, demonstrated inhibition of radiographic progression in RA patients.

5.2.4 Figlotinib

Filgotinib presents a selectivity of almost 30-fold for JAK1 versus JAK2, with dose-dependent inhibition of Th1-Th2 [124, 130]. The most frequent side effects reported for JAK1 selective inhibitors are represented by nausea, cephalalgia, respiratory and urinary infections, dose-related neutropenia and an increase in serum levels for creatinine and hepatic enzymes [127].

6. Conclusions

The extensive research of the last two decades has concerned the diagnosis and individual prognosis of patients with RA and also the elaboration of personal treatment strategies.

Case management requires a continuous evaluation of the risk/benefit ratio of the therapy, so that the results are optimal and with minimal adverse effects and complications, including infections.

Also, anticipating a balance between the risks of comorbidities and the benefits of treatment is a management strategy that must be taken into account.

Conflict of interest

The authors declare no conflict of interest.

Author details

Mihail Virgil Boldeanu[1†], Adrian Răzvan Ionescu[2†], Valeriu Horaţiu Popoviciu[3†], Andreea Lili Bărbulescu[4†], Ştefan Cristian Dinescu[4†], Isabela Siloşi[1†], Maria Forţofoiu[5†], Rodica Pădureanu[6†], Andreea Meca[6†], Vlad Pădureanu[7†], Mircea Cătălin Forţofoiu[7†], Ioan Sabin Poenariu[6†], Lidia Boldeanu[8*†] and Ananu Florentin Vreju[4†]

1 Faculty of Medicine, Department of Immunology, University of Medicine and Pharmacy of Craiova, Craiova, Romania

2 Faculty of Medicine, Department 5 Internal Medicine, "Carol Davila" University of Medicine and Pharmacy, Bucharest, Romania

3 Faculty of Medicine, Department of Rheumatology, University of Medicine, Pharmacy, Science and Technology of Târgu Mureş, Romania

4 Faculty of Medicine, Department of Rheumatology, University of Medicine and Pharmacy of Craiova, Craiova, Romania

5 Faculty of Medicine, Department of Emergency Medicine and First Aid, University of Medicine and Pharmacy of Craiova, Craiova, Romania

6 University of Medicine and Pharmacy of Craiova, Craiova, Romania

7 Faculty of Medicine, Department of Internal Medicine, University of Medicine and Pharmacy of Craiova, Craiova, Romania

8 Faculty of Medicine, Department of Microbiology, University of Medicine and Pharmacy of Craiova, Craiova, Romania

*Address all correspondence to: barulidia@yahoo.com

† All authors made an equal contribution to the paper, to that of first authors, and thus share the main authorship.

References

[1] Padyukov L, Seielstad M, Ong RT, Ding B, Ronnelid J, Seddighzadeh M, et al. A genome-wide association study suggests contrasting associations in ACPA-positive versus ACPA-negative rheumatoid arthritis. Annals of the Rheumatic Diseases. 2011;**70**(2):259-265. DOI: 10.1136/ard.2009.126821

[2] Schellekens GA, Visser H, de Jong BA, van den Hoogen FH, Hazes JM, Breedveld FC, et al. The diagnostic properties of rheumatoid arthritis antibodies recognizing a cyclic citrullinated peptide. Arthritis and Rheumatism. 2000;**43**(1):155-163

[3] Guo Q, Wang Y, Xu D, Nossent J, Pavlos NJ, Xu J. Rheumatoid arthritis: Pathological mechanisms and modern pharmacologic therapies. Bone Research. 2018;**6**:15. DOI: 10.1038/s41413-018-0016-9

[4] Wang Z, Nicholls SJ, Rodriguez ER, Kummu O, Hörkkö S, Barnard J, et al. Protein carbamylation links inflammation, smoking, uremia and atherogenesis. Nature Medicine. 2007;**13**(10):1176-1184

[5] Svendsen AJ, Junker P, Houen G, Kyvik KO, Nielsen C, Skytthe A, et al. Incidence of chronic persistent rheumatoid arthritis and the impact of smoking: A historical twin cohort study. Arthritis Care & Research (Hoboken). 2017;**69**(5):616-624. DOI: 10.1002/acr.22987

[6] Klareskog L, Stolt P, Lundberg K, Källberg H, Bengtsson C, Grunewald J, et al. A new model for an etiology of rheumatoid arthritis: Smoking may trigger HLA-DR (shared epitope)-restricted immune reactions to autoantigens modified by citrullination. Arthritis and Rheumatism. 2006;**54**(1):38-46

[7] Villanueva-Romero R, Gutiérrez-Cañas I, Carrión M, Pérez-García S, Seoane IV, Martínez C, et al. The anti-inflammatory mediator, vasoactive intestinal peptide, modulates the differentiation and function of Th subsets in rheumatoid arthritis. Journal of Immunology Research. 2018;**2018**:6043710. DOI: 10.1155/2018/6043710

[8] Calabresi E, Petrelli F, Bonifacio AF, Puxeddu I, Alunno A. One year in review 2018: Pathogenesis of rheumatoid arthritis. Clinical and Experimental Rheumatology. 2018;**36**(2):175-184

[9] Sherina N, Hreggvidsdottir HS, Bengtsson C, Hansson M, Israelsson L, Alfredsson L, et al. Low levels of antibodies against common viruses associate with anti-citrullinated protein antibody-positive rheumatoid arthritis; implications for disease aetiology. Arthritis Research & Therapy. 2017;**19**(1):219. DOI: 10.1186/s13075-017-1423-9

[10] Chiang HI, Li JR, Liu CC, Liu PY, Chen HH, Chen YM, et al. An association of gut microbiota with different phenotypes in Chinese patients with rheumatoid arthritis. Journal of Clinical Medicine. 2019;**8**(11):E1770. DOI: 10.3390/jcm8111770

[11] Kishikawa T, Maeda Y, Nii T, Motooka D, Matsumoto Y, Matsushita M, et al. Metagenome-wide association study of gut microbiome revealed novel aetiology of rheumatoid arthritis in the Japanese population. Annals of the Rheumatic Diseases. 2020;**79**(1):103-111. DOI: 10.1136/annrheumdis-2019-215743

[12] Radić M. Role of helicobacter pylori infection in autoimmune systemic rheumatic diseases. World Journal of

Gastroenterology. 2014;**20**(36):12839-12846. DOI: 10.3748/wjg.v20.i36.12839

[13] Joo YB, Lim YH, Kim KJ, Park KS, Park YJ. Respiratory viral infections and the risk of rheumatoid arthritis. Arthritis Research & Therapy. 2019;**21**(1):199. DOI: 10.1186/s13075-019-1977-9

[14] Yarwood A, Huizinga TWJ, Worthington J. The genetics of rheumatoid arthritis: Risk and protection in different stages of the evolution of RA. Rheumatology (Oxford, England). 2014;**55**(2):199-209. DOI: 10.1093/rheumatology/keu323

[15] Hensvold AH, Magnusson PK, Joshua V, Hansson M, Israelsson L, Ferreira R, et al. Environmental and genetic factors in the development of anticitrullinated protein antibodies (ACPAs) and ACPA-positive rheumatoid arthritis: An epidemiological investigation in twins. Annals of the Rheumatic Diseases. 2015;**74**(2):375-380. DOI: 10.1136/annrheumdis-2013-203947

[16] Bos WH, Ursum J, de Vries N, Bartelds GM, Wolbink GJ, Nurmohamed MT, et al. The role of the shared epitope in arthralgia with anti-cyclic citrullinated peptide antibodies (anti-CCP), and its effect on anti-CCP levels. Annals of the Rheumatic Diseases. 2008;**67**(9):1347-1350. DOI: 10.1136/ard.2008.089953

[17] Lin L, Chen Y, Xiao Z, Huang S, Yang Z. The association of HLA-DRB1 alleles with rheumatoid arthritis in the Chinese Shantou population: A follow-up study. Biochemistry and Cell Biology. 2007;**85**(2):227-238. DOI: 10.1139/o06-204

[18] Mattey DL, Dawes PT, Clarke S, Fisher J, Brownfield A, Thomson W, et al. Relationship among the HLA-DRB1 shared epitope, smoking, and rheumatoid factor production in rheumatoid arthritis. Arthritis and Rheumatism. 2002;**47**(4):403-407. DOI: 10.1002/art.10514

[19] van der Woude D, Houwing-Duistermaat JJ, Toes RE, Huizinga TW, Thomson W, Worthington J, et al. Quantitative heritability of anti-citrullinated protein antibody-positive and anti-citrullinated protein antibody-negative rheumatoid arthritis. Arthritis and Rheumatism. 2009;**60**(4):916-923. DOI: 10.1002/art.24385

[20] van der Woude D, Lie BA, Lundstrom E, Balsa A, Feitsma AL, Houwing-Duistermaat JJ, et al. Protection against anti-citrullinated protein antibody-positive rheumatoid arthritis is predominantly associated with HLA-DRB1*1301: A meta-analysis of HLA-DRB1 associations with anti-citrullinated protein antibody-positive and anti-citrullinated protein antibody-negative rheumatoid arthritis in four European populations. Arthritis and Rheumatism. 2010;**62**(5):1236-1245. DOI: 10.1002/art.27366

[21] Plant D, Thomson W, Lunt M, Flynn E, Martin P, Eyre S, et al. The role of rheumatoid arthritis genetic susceptibility markers in the prediction of erosive disease in patients with early inflammatory polyarthritis: Results from the Norfolk arthritis register. Rheumatology (Oxford, England). 2011;**50**(1):78-84. DOI: 10.1093/rheumatology/keq032

[22] Bizzaro N, Bartoloni E, Morozzi G, Manganelli S, Riccieri V, Sabatini P, et al. Anti-cyclic citrullinated peptide antibody titer predicts time to rheumatoid arthritis onset in patients with undifferentiated arthritis: results from a 2-year prospective study. Arthritis Research & Therapy. 2013;**15**(1):R16. DOI: 10.1186/ar4148

[23] Hueber AJ, Asquith DL, Miller AM, Reilly J, Kerr S, Leipe J, et al. Mast cells express IL-17A in rheumatoid arthritis synovium. Journal of Immunology. 2010;**184**(7):3336-3340. DOI: 10.4049/jimmunol.0903566

[24] Pratt AG, Isaacs JD. Seronegative rheumatoid arthritis: Pathogenetic and therapeutic aspects. Best Practice & Research. Clinical Rheumatology. 2014;**28**(4):651-659. DOI: 10.1016/j.berh.2014.10.016

[25] Molendijk M, Hazes JM, Lubberts E. From patients with arthralgia, pre-RA and recently diagnosed RA: What is the current status of understanding RA pathogenesis. RMD Open. 2018;**4**(1):e000256. DOI: 10.1136/rmdopen-2016-000256

[26] Hill Gaston JS. Cellular immunity in rheumatoid arthritis. In: Hochberg MC, Silman AJ, Smolen JS, Weinblatt ME, Weisman MH, editors. Rheumatology. 6th ed. China: Mosby; 2015. pp. 758-763

[27] van den Berg WB, Miossec P. IL-17 as a future therapeutic target for rheumatoid arthritis. Nature Reviews Rheumatology. 2009;**5**(10):549-553. DOI: 10.1038/nrrheum.2009.179

[28] Szekanecz Z, Besenyei T, Paragh G, Koch AE. Angiogenesis in rheumatoid arthritis. Autoimmunity. 2009;**42**(7):563-573. DOI: 10.1080/08916930903143083

[29] Marrelli A, Cipriani P, Liakouli V, Carubbi F, Perricone C, Perricone R, et al. Angiogenesis in rheumatoid arthritis: A disease specific process or a common response to chronic inflammation? Autoimmunity Reviews. 2011;**10**(10):595-598. DOI: 10.1016/j.autrev.2011.04.020

[30] Wojdasiewicz P, Wajda A, Haładyj E, Romanowska-Próchnicka K, Felis-Giemza A, Nałęcz-Janik J, et al. IL-35, TNF-α, BAFF, and VEGF serum levels in patients with different rheumatic diseases. Reumatologia. 2019;**57**(3):145-150. DOI: 10.5114/reum.2019.86424

[31] Tweehuysen L, van den Ende CH, Beeren FM, Been EM, van den Hoogen FH, den Broeder AA. Little evidence for usefulness of biomarkers for predicting successful dose reduction or discontinuation of a biologic agent in rheumatoid arthritis. Arthritis & Rheumatology. 2017;**69**(2):301-308. DOI: 10.1002/art.39946

[32] Harre U, Georgess D, Bang H, Bozec A, Axmann R, Ossipova E, et al. Induction of osteoclastogenesis and bone loss by human autoantibodies against citrullinated vimentin. The Journal of Clinical Investigation. 2012;**122**(5):1791-1802. DOI: 10.1172/JCI60975

[33] Turesson C, Matteson EL. Extraarticular features of rheumatoid arthritis and systemic involvement. In: Hochberg MC, Silman AJ, Smolen JS, Weinblatt ME, Weisman MH, editors. Rheumatology. 6th ed. China: Mosby; 2015. pp. 712-719

[34] Aletaha D, Neogi T, Silman AJ, Funovits J, Felson DT, Bingham CO 3rd, et al. 2010 rheumatoid arthritis classification criteria: an American College of Rheumatology/European Ligue Against Rheumatism collaborative initiative. Annals of the Rheumatic Diseases. 2010;**69**(9):1580-1588. DOI: 10.1136/ard.2010.138461

[35] Mueller RB, Kaegi T, Haile SR, Schulze-Koops H, Schiff M, von Kempis J. Clinical and radiographic course of early undifferentiated arthritis under treatment is not dependent on the number of joints with erosions at diagnosis: Results from the Swiss prospective observational cohort. RMD Open. 2018;**4**(1):e000673. DOI: 10.1136/rmdopen-2018-000673

[36] Kung T, Bykerk V. Detecting the earliest signs of rheumatoid arthritis: Symptoms and examination. Rheumatic Diseases Clinics of North America. 2014;**40**(4):669-683. DOI: 10.1016/j.rdc.2014.07.009

[37] Holers VM. Insights from populations at risk for the furture development of classified rheumatoid arthritis. Rheumatic Diseases Clinics of North America. 2014;**40**(4):605-620. DOI: 10.1016/j.rdc.2014.07.003

[38] Sparks JA. Rheumatoid arthritis. Annals of Internal Medicine. 2019;**170**(1):ITC1-ITC16. DOI: 10.7326/AITC201901010

[39] Stack RJ, Sahni M, Mallen CD, Raza K. Symptom complexes at the earliest phases of rheumatoid arthritis: A symthesis of the qualitative literature. Arthritis Care & Research (Hoboken). 2013;**65**(12):1916-1926. DOI: 10.1002/acr.22097

[40] Williams G. The genesis of chronic illness: Narrative re-construction. Sociology of Health & Illness. 1984;**6**(2):175-200

[41] Griffith J, Carr A. What is the impact of, early rheumatoid arthritis on the individual? Best Practice & Research. Clinical Rheumatology. 2001;**15**(1):77-90

[42] Lempp H, Scott D, Kingsley G. The personal impact of rheumatoid arthritis on patients' identity: A qualitative study. Chronic Illness. 2006;**2**(2):109-120

[43] Kumar K, Daley E, Khattak F, Buckley CD, Raza K. The influence of ethnicity on the extent of, and reasons underlying, delay in general practitioner consultation in patients with RA. Rheumatology (Oxford). 2010;**49**(50):1005-1012. DOI: 10.1093/rheumatology/keq011

[44] Oliver S, Bosworth A, Airoldi M, Bunyan H, Callum A, Dixon J, et al. Exploring the healthcare journey of patients with rheumatoid arthritis: A mapping project. Implications for practice. Musculoskeletal Care. 2008;**6**(4):247-266. DOI: 10.1002/msc.139

[45] Bury M. Chronic illness as biographical disruption. Sociology of Health & Illness. 1982;**4**(2):167-182

[46] Neil J. Transcendence and transformation in the life patterns of women living with rheumatoid arthritis. ANS. Advances in Nursing Science. 2002;**24**(4):27-47

[47] Sheppard J, Kumar K, Buckley CD, Shaw KL, Raza K. "I just thought it was normal aches and pains": A qualitative study of decision-making processes in patients with early rheumatoid arthritis. Rheumatology (Oxford, England). 2008;**47**(10):1577-1582. DOI: 10.1093/rheumatology/ken304

[48] Townsend A, Adam P, Cox SM, Li LC. Everyday ethics and help-seeking in early rheumatoid arthritis. Chronic Illness. 2010;**6**(3):171-182. DOI: 10.1177/1742395309351963

[49] Bury M. Meanings at risk: The experience of arthritis. In: Anderson R, Bury M, editors. Living with Chronic Ilnness. London: Unwin Hyman; 1988. pp. 89-116

[50] Wiener CL. The burden of rheumatoid arthritis: Tolerating the uncertainty. Social Science & Medicine. 1975;**9**(2):97-104. DOI: 10.1016/0037-7856(75)90101-8

[51] Backman CL, Smith LF, Smith S, Montie PL, Suto M. Experience of mothers living with inflammatory arthritis. Arthritis and Rheumatism. 2007;**57**(3):381-388

[52] Williams AE, Graham AS. "My feet: Visible, but ignored ...". A qualitative study of foot care for people with rheumatoid arthritis. Clinical Rehabilitation. 2012;**26**(10):952-959. DOI: 10.1177/0269215511434995

[53] Nyman CS, Lutzen K. Caring needs of patients with rheumatoid arthritis. Nursing Science Quarterly. 1999;**12**(2):164-169

[54] Brown S, Williams A. Women's experiences of rheumatoid arthritis. Journal of Advanced Nursing. 1995;**21**(4):695-701

[55] Shaul MP. Transitions in chronic illness: Rheumatoid arthritis in women. Rehabilitation Nursing. 1997;**22**(4):199-205

[56] Hewlett S, Cockshott Z, Byron M, Kitchen K, Tipler S, Pope D, et al. Patients' perceptions of fatigue in rheumatoid arthritis: Overwhelming, uncontrollable, ignored. Arthritis and Rheumatism. 2005;**53**(5):697-702

[57] Stamm T, Lovelock L, Stew G, Nell V, Smolen J, Jonsson H, et al. I have mastered the challenge of living with a chronic disease: Life stories of people with rheumatoid arthritis. Qualitative Health Research. 2008;**18**(5):658-669. DOI: 10.1177/1049732308316348

[58] Bernatsky S, Feldman D, De Civita M, Haggerty J, Tousignant P, Legaré J, et al. Optimal care for rheumatoid arthritis: A focus group study. Clinical Rheumatology. 2010;**29**(6):645-657. DOI: 10.1007/s10067-010-1383-9

[59] Sakalys JA. Illness behavior in rheumatoid arthritis. Arthritis Care and Research. 1997;**10**:229-237

[60] Yoshida K. Uncertainty in the lives of people with spinal cord injury and rheumatoid arthritis. Canadian Journal of Rehabilitation. 1996;**10**:5-14

[61] Fair BS. Contrasts in patients' and providers' explanations of rheumatoid arthritis. Journal of Nursing Scholarship. 2003;**35**(4):339-344

[62] Zhao J, Su Y, Li R, Ye H, Zou Q, Fang Y, et al. Classification criteria of early rheumatoid arthritis and validation of its performance in a multi-center cohort. Clinical and Experimental Rheumatology. 2014;**32**(5):667-673

[63] Hua C, Daien CI, Combe B, Landewe R. Diagnosis, prognosis and classification of early arthritis: Results of a systematic review informing the 2016 update of the EULAR recommendations for the management of early arthritis. RMD Open. 2017;**3**(1):e000406. DOI: 10.1136/rmdopen-2016-000406

[64] Combe B, Landewe R, Daien CI, Hua C, Aletaha D, Álvaro-Gracia JM, et al. 2016 update of the EULAR recommendations for the management of early arthritis. Annals of the Rheumatic Diseases. 2017;**76**(6):948-959. DOI: 10.1136/annrheumdis-2016-210602

[65] Mankia K, Emery P. Preclinical rheumatoid arthritis. Arthritis & Rhematology. 2016;**68**(4):779-788. DOI: 10.1002/art.39603

[66] Brasington R. Clinical features of rheumatoid arthritis. In: Hochberg M, Silman A, Smolen J, Weinblatt M, Weisman M, editors. Rheumatology. 4th ed. Vol. 2. Mosby Elsevier; 2008. pp. 763-771

[67] Trieb K. Treatment of the wrist in rheumatoid arthritis. The Journal of Hand Surgery. 2008;**33**(1):113-123. DOI: 10.1016/j.jhsa.2007.09.011

[68] Johnsson PM, Eberhardt K. Hand deformities are important signs of disease severity in patients with early rheumatoid arthritis. Rheumatology (Oxford, England). 2009;**48**(11):1398-1401. DOI: 10.1093/rheumatology/kep253

[69] Coons MS, Green SM. Boutonniere deformity. Hand Clinics. 1995;**11**(3):387-402

[70] Ridley WE, Xiang H, Han J, Ridley LJ. Swan neck deformity. Journal of Medical Imaging and Radiation Oncology. 2018;**62**(Suppl 1):159-160. DOI: 10.1111/1754-9485.31_12786

[71] Monreal R. Extensor Indicis Proprius Tenodesis to correct finger ulnar drift deformity in rheumatoid arthritis. Hand. 2016;**11**(3):336-340

[72] Shinagawa S, Okamura K, Yonemoto Y, Shitara H, Suto T, Sakane H, et al. Shoulder tenderness was associated with the inflammatory changes on magnetic resonance imaging in patients with rheumatoid arthritis. Scientific Reports. 2019;**9**(1):19599. DOI: 10.1038/s41598-019-55938-6

[73] Papadakis M, Manios A, Trompoukis C. Popliteal cyst before William baker: First report in the Galenic corpus. Acta Chirurgica Belgica. 2017;**117**(2):131-134. DOI: 10.1080/00015458.2017.1289734

[74] Görtz S, Fricka K, Bugbee W. The hip. In: Hochberg M, Silman A, Smolen J, Weinblatt M, Weisman M, editors. Rheumatology. 6th ed. Vol. 1. China: Mosby; 2015. pp. 626-632

[75] Gutierrez M, Pineda C, Salaffi F, Raffeiner B, Cazenave T, Martinez-Nava GA, et al. Is ankle involvement underestimated in rheumatoid arthritis? Results of a multicenter ultrasound study. Clinical Rheumatology. 2016;**35**(11):2669-2678

[76] Turesson C, Matteson E. Extra-articular features of rheumatoid arthritis and systemic involvement. In: Hochberg M, Silman A, Smolen J, Weinblatt M, Weisman M, editors. Rheumatology. 4th ed. Vol. 2. Mosby Elsevier; 2008. pp. 773-783

[77] Ciurea P. Medicina Interna-Reumatologie. Craiova: Ed. Medicala Universitara; 2013. pp. 123-153

[78] Balint GP, Balint PV. Felty's syndrome. Best Practice & Research. Clinical Rheumatology. 2004;**18**(5):631-645. DOI: 10.1016/j.berh.2004.05.002

[79] Tanoue LT. Pulmonary manifestation of rheumatoid arthritis. Clinics in Chest Medicine. 1998;**19**(4):667-685

[80] Hara KS, Ballard DJ, Ilstrum DM, Connolly DC, Vollertsen RS. Rheumatoid pericarditis: Clinical features and survival. Medicine. 1990;**69**(2):81-91

[81] Voskuyl AE. The heart and cardiovascular manifestations in rheumatoid arthritis. Rheumatology (Oxford). 2006;**45**(Suppl 4):iv4-iv7

[82] Bolosiu HD. Osteoporoza-Ghid de Studiu. Cluj Napoca: Editura UMF; 2002

[83] Sharp JT, Lidsky MD, Collins LC, Moreland J. Methods of scoring the progression of radiologic changes in rheumatoid arthritis: Correlation of radiologic, clinical and laboratory abnormalities. Arthritis and Rheumatism. 1971;**14**(6):706-720. DOI: 10.1002/art.1780140605

[84] van der Heijde D. How to read radiographs according to the Sharp/van der Heijde method. The Journal of Rheumatology. 2000;**27**(1):261-263

[85] Learch T. Imaging of rheumatoid arthritis. In: Hochberg M, Silman A, Smolen J, Weinblatt M, Weisman M,

editors. Rheumatology. 4th ed. Vol. 2. Mosby Elsevier; 2008. pp. 763-793-800

[86] Lindqvist E, Jonsson K, Saxne T, Eberhardt K. Course of radiographic damage over 10 years in a cohort with early rheumatoid arthritis. Annals of the Rheumatic Diseases. 2003;**62**:611-616. DOI: 10.1136/ard.62.7.611

[87] Kloppenburg M, Kroon FP, Blanco FJ, Doherty M, Dziedzic KS, Greibrokk E, et al. 2018 update of the EULAR recommendations for the management of hand osteoarthritis. Annals of the Rheumatic Diseases. 2019;**78**(1):16-24. DOI: 10.1136/annrheumdis-2018-213826

[88] Bouchaud-Chabot A, Liote F. Cervical spine involvement in rheumatoid arthritis. A review. Joint Bone Spine. 2002;**69**(2):141-154

[89] Neva MH, Kaarela K, Kauppi M. Prevalence of radiological changes in the cervical spine-a cross-sectional study after 20 years from presentation of rheumatoid arthritis. The Journal of Rheumatology. 2000;**27**(1):90-93

[90] Colebatch A, Edwards CJ, Østergaard M, van der Heijde D, Balint PV, D'Agostino MA, et al. EULAR recommendations for the use of imaging of the joints in the clinical management of rheumatoid arthritis. Annals of the Rheumatic Diseases. 2013;**72**(6):804-814. DOI: 10.1136/annrheumdis-2012-203158

[91] Barbulescu AL, Ciurea PL, Mitran C, Chisalau BA, Parvanescu CD, Firulescu SC, et al. High frequency ultrasonography of the hand versus anti-RA33 evaluation in early rheumatoid arthritis - A pilot study. Medical Ultrasonography. 2017;**19**(2):166-171. DOI: 10.11152/mu-995

[92] Vreju FA, Ciurea PL, Rosu A, Chisalau BA, Parvanescu CD, Firulescu SC, et al. The effect of glucosamine, chondroitin and harpagophytum procumbens on femoral hyaline cartilage thickness in patients with knee osteoarthritis- an MRI versus ultrasonography study. Journal of Mind and Medical Sciences. 2019;**6**(1):162-168

[93] Vreju FA, Filippucci E, Gutierrez M, Di Geso L, Ciapetti A, Ciurea ME, et al. Subclinical ultrasound synovitis in a particular joint is associated with ultrasound evidence of bone erosions in that same joint in rheumatoid patients in clinical remission. Clinical and Experimental Rheumatology. 2016;**34**(4):673-678

[94] Backhaus M, Burmester GR, Sandrock D, Loreck D, Hess D, Scholz A, et al. Prospective two year follow up study comparing novel and conventional imaging procedures in patients with arthritic finger joints. Annals of the Rheumatic Diseases. 2002;**61**(10):895-904

[95] Wakefield RJ, Balint PV, Szkudlarek M, Filippucci E, Backhaus M, D'gostino MA, et al. Conaghan PG; OMERACT 7 special interest group. OMERACT 7 special interest group musculoskeletal ultrasound including definitions for ultrasonographic pathology. The Journal of Rheumatology. 2006;**32**(12):2485-2487

[96] Døhn UM, Terslev L, Szkudlarek M, Hansen MS, Hetland ML, Hansen A, et al. Detection, scoring and volume assessment of bone erosions by ultrasonography in rheumatoid arthritis: Comparison with CT. Annals of the Rheumatic Diseases. 2013;**72**(4):530-534. DOI: 10.1136/annrheumdis-2011-201114

[97] D'Agostino MA, Terslev L, Aegerter P, Backhaus M, Balint P, Bruyn GA, et al. Scoring ultrasound synovitis in rheumatoid arthritis: A EULAR - OMERACT ultrasound

taskforce - part 1: Definition and development of a standardized, consensus-based scoring system. RMD Open. 2017;**3**(1):e000428. DOI: 10.1136/rmdopen-2016-000428

[98] Gutierrez M, Filippucci E, Ruta S, Ruta S, Salaffi F, Blasetti P, et al. Inter-observer reliability of high-resolution ultrasonography in the assessment of bone erosions in patients with rheumatoid arthritis: Experience of an intensive dedicated training programme. Rheumatology (Oxford, England). 2011;**50**(2):373-380. DOI: 10.1093/rheumatology/keq320

[99] Ammitzbøll-Danielsen M, Østergaard M, Naredo E, Terslev L. Validity and sensitivity to change of the semi-quantitative OMERACT ultrasound scoring system for tenosynovitis in patients with rheumatoid arthritis. Rheumatology (Oxford, England). 2016;**55**(12):2156-2166. DOI: 10.1093/rheumatology/kew317

[100] Terslev L, Østergaard M, Sexton J, Hammer HB. Is synovial hypertrophy without Doppler activity sensitive to change? Post-hoc analysis from a rheumatoid arthritis ultrasound study. Arthritis Research & Therapy. 2018;**20**:224. DOI: 10.1186/s13075-018-1709-6

[101] Nam JL, Hensor EM, Hunt L, Conaghan PG, Wakefield RJ, Emery P. Ultrasound findings predict progression to inflammatory arthritis in anti-CCP antibody-positive patients without clinical synovitis. Annals of the Rheumatic Diseases. 2016;**75**(12):2060-2067

[102] van der Ven M, van der Veer-Meerkerk M, Ten Cate DF, Rasappu N, Kok MR, Csakvari D, et al. Absence of ultrasound inflammation in patients presenting with arthralgia rules out the development of arthritis. Arthritis Research & Therapy. 2017;**19**(1):202. DOI: 10.1186/s13075-017-1405-y

[103] Brown AK, Conaghan PG, Karim Z, Quinn MA, Ikeda K, Peterfy CG, et al. An explanation for the apparent dissociation between clinical remission and continued structural deterioration in rheumatoid arthritis. Arthritis and Rheumatism. 2008;**58**(10):2958-2967. DOI: 10.1002/art.23945

[104] Saleem B, Brown AK, Keen H, Nizam S, Freeston J, Wakefield R, et al. Should imaging be a component of rheumatoid arthritis remission criteria? A comparison between traditional and modified composite remission scores and imaging assessments. Annals of the Rheumatic Diseases. 2011;**70**(5):792-798. DOI: 10.1136/ard.2010.134445

[105] D'Agostino MA, Padovano I, Iagnocco A. Imaging. In: Bijlsma J, Hachulla E, editors. Textbook on rheumatic diseases. 3rd ed. Ed. BMJ Publishing Groupt Ltd; 2018. pp. 122-157

[106] Smolen JS, Landewé RBM, Bijlsma JWJ, et al. EULAR recommendations for the management of rheumatoid arthritis with synthetic and biological disease-modifying antirheumatic drugs: 2019 update. Annals of the Rheumatic Diseases. 2020;**0**:1-15. DOI: 10.1136/annrheumdis-2019-216655

[107] DiPiro JT, Talbert RL, Yee GC, Matzke GR, Wells BG, Posey LM. Pharmacotherapy: A Pathophysiologic Approach. 10th ed. McGraw-Hill Education; 2016. pp. 4034-4076

[108] Bonifacio AF, Alunno A, La Paglia GMC, Valentini E, Leone MC, Bartoloni E, et al. Novel autoantibodies in rheumatoid arthritis. Reumatismo. 2019;**71**(1):1-12. DOI: 10.4081/reumatismo.2019.1102

[109] Whittlesea C, Hodson K. Clinical Pharmacy and Therapeutics. 6th ed. Elsevier; 2019. pp. 923-948

[110] Ziarko M, Siemiatkowska K, Sienski M, Samborski W, Samborska J, Mojs E. Mental health and rheumatoid arthritis: Toward understanding the emotional status of people with chronic disease. BioMed Research International. 2019;**2019**:1473925. DOI: 10.1155/2019/1473925

[111] Kurata I, Tsuboi H, Terasaki M, Shimizu M, Toko H, Honda F, et al. Effect of biological disease-modifying anti-rheumatic drugs on airway and interstitial lung disease in patients with rheumatoid arthritis. Internal Medicine. 2019;**58**(12):1703-1712. DOI: 10.2169/internalmedicine.2226-18

[112] Watanabe T, Fukae J, Fukaya S, Sawamukai N, Isobe M, Matsuhashi M, et al. Incidence and risk factors for reactivation from resolved hepatitis B virus in rheumatoid arthritis patients treated with biological disease-modifying antirheumatic drugs. International Journal of Rheumatic Diseases. 2019;**22**(4):574-582. DOI: 10.1111/1756-185X.13401

[113] Ho CTK, Mok CC, Cheung TT, Kwok KY, Yip RML. Hong Kong society of rheumatology. Clinical Rheumatology. 2019;**38**(12):3331-3350. DOI: 10.1007/s10067-019-04761-5

[114] Available from: https://www.ema.europa.eu/en/documents/product-information/humira-epar-product-information_en.pdf

[115] Al-Salama ZT. FKB327: An Adalimumab biosimilar. BioDrugs. 2019;**33**(1):113-116. DOI: 10.1007/s40259-019-00335-8

[116] Available from: https://www.ema.europa.eu/en/documents/product-information/enbrel-epar-product-information_en.pdf

[117] Pelechas E, Drosos AA. Etanercept biosimilar SB-4. Expert Opinion on Biological Therapy. 2019;**19**(3):173-179. DOI: 10.1080/14712598.2019.1566456

[118] Available from: https://www.ema.europa.eu/en/documents/assessment-report/simponi-epar-public-assessment-report_en.pdf

[119] Available from: https://www.ema.europa.eu/en/documents/product-information/orencia-epar-product-information_en.pdf

[120] Choquette D, Bessette L, Alemao E, Haraoui B, Postema R, Raynauld JP, et al. Persistence rates of abatacept and TNF inhibitors used as first or second biologic DMARDs in the treatment of rheumatoid arthritis: 9 years of experience from the Rhumadata® clinical database and registry. Arthritis Research & Therapy. 2019;**21**(1):138. DOI: 10.1186/s13075-019-1917-8

[121] González-Fernández MA, Villamañán E, Jiménez-Nácher I, Moreno F, Herrero A, Balsa A. Persistence of biological agents over an eight-year period in rheumatoid arthritis and spondyloarthritis patients. Farmacia Hospitalaria. 2019;**43**(1):24-30. DOI: 10.7399/fh.11080

[122] Available from: https://www.ema.europa.eu/en/documents/product-information/roactemra-epar-product-information_en.pdf

[123] Available from: https://www.ema.europa.eu/en/documents/product-information/kineret-epar-product-information_en.pdf

[124] Silvagni E, Di Battista M, Bonifacio AF, Zucchi D, Governato G, Scire CA. One year in review 2019: Novelties in the treatment of rheumatoid arthritis. Clinical and Experimental Rheumatology. 2019;**37**:519-534

[125] Choy EH. Clinical significance of janus kinase inhibitor selectivity. Rheumatology (Oxford, England). 2019;**58**(6):953-962

[126] Hodge JA, Kawabata TT, Krinshnaswami S, Clrk JD, Telliez JB, Dowty ME, et al. The mechanism of action of tofacitinib-an oral Janus kinase inhibitor for the treatment of rheumatoid arthritis. Clinical and Experimental Rheumatology. 2016;**34**:318-328

[127] Rigby WFC, Lampl K, Low MJ, Frust DE. Review of routine laboratory monitoring for patients with rheumatoid arthritis receiving biologic or nonbiologic DMARDs. International Journal of Rheumatology. 2017;**2017**:9614241. DOI: 10.1155/2017/9614241

[128] Mogul A, Corsi K, McAuliffe L. Baricitinib: The second FDA-approved JAK inhibitor for the treatment of rheumatoid arthritis. The Annals of Pharmacotherapy. 2019;**53**(9):947-953

[129] Olumiant 2 mg and 4 mg film-coated tablets. SPC. Available from: http://www.ema.europa.eu/docs/en_GB/document_library/EPAR_-_Product_Information/human/004085/WC500223723

[130] Biggioggero M, Becciolini A, Crotii C, Agape E, Favali EG. Upadacitinib and filgotinib: the role of JAK1 selective inhibition in the treatment of rheumatoid arthritis. Drugs in Context. 2019;**24**(8):212595. DOI: 10.7573/dic.212595

Chapter 7

Self-Management in Patients with Rheumatoid Arthritis

Wen Luo, Xiuli Zhang and Kaijing Ren

Abstract

Despite the effective pharmacological management of the disease over the last two decades, many individuals with RA continue to have psychological distress, and this is associated with poor outcomes. Addressing psychological issues hand in hand with pharmacological treatment will help to maximize outcomes for people with RA. Self-management (SM) is of utmost importance for people with rheumatoid arthritis to minimize their complaints, reduce clinic visits, and reduce disability. Considering the continuous update on the guidelines for disease management, non-pharmacological management remains a poorly addressed need of importance. In this chapter, we will introduce the current and progress of self-management in patients with rheumatoid arthritis.

Keywords: rheumatoid arthritis, self-management, self-efficacy, patient education

1. Introduction

Rheumatoid arthritis (RA) is a severe chronic disabling disease, characterized by joint pain and inflammation as the physical symptoms [1]. Disease-related functional damage with limited mobility of the affected joints, significantly decline patients' quality of life [2]. Although medical treatment is an integral part in rheumatoid arthritis, this disease has a major impact on patients' life. Patients with rheumatoid arthritis are classically influenced by five factors according to the International Classification of Functioning (ICF): physical function, body activities, participation, individual factors, and environmental factors [3]. During the past two decades, self-management (SM) strategies have been emphasized to help patients with rheumatoid arthritis cope with the incapacitating symptoms of the disease [4].

There are many different definitions of self-management worldwide. Now most researchers in various fields accept Lorig's definition, that is, self-management refers to a kind of healthy behavior that maintains and improves one's own health through the behavior of patients; heals and manages the symptoms and symptoms of one's own diseases; reduces the influence of diseases on one's own social functions, emotions, and interpersonal relationships; and persistently treats one's own diseases. The latest theoretical study is the individual family self-management theory proposed by Polly Ryan of the University of Wisconsin. The theory defines self-management behavior as a complex phenomenon with internal motivation, including context, process, and outcome. The situational part includes special situational factors, environmental factors, and personal family factors. The special situational factors consist of treatment, stability, and recovery of the disease.

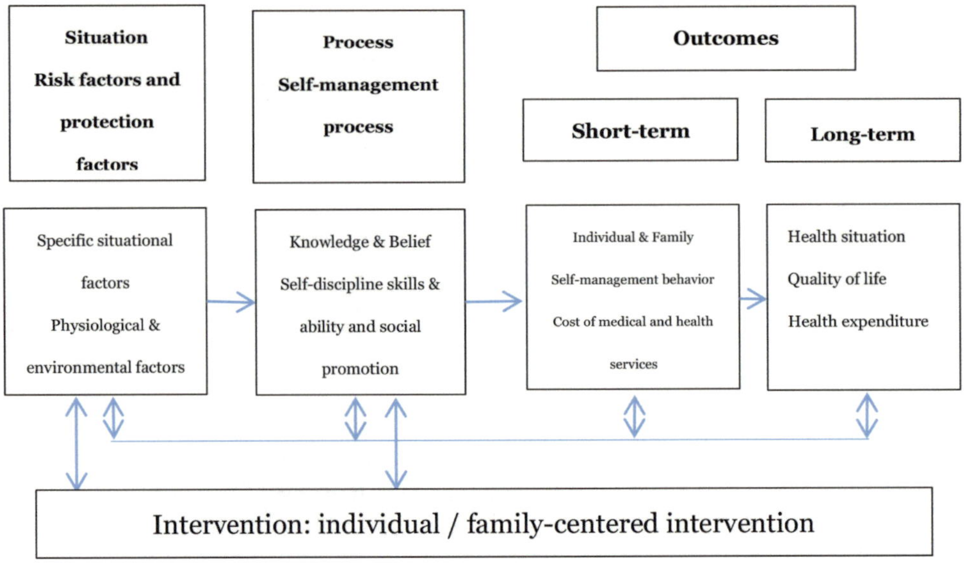

Figure 1.
Theoretical framework of individual and family self-management.

The environmental factors include the access and transfer channels of medical resources, transportation, surrounding environment, work, and culture. The individual/family factors include individual development stage, language level, information processing mode, and ability. The process gets into knowledge and belief, for example, self-efficacy. The outcomes include the behavior change, symptom management, and drug treatment. The short-term outcomes consist of treatment and healthcare costs. The long-term outcomes include health status, quality of life, and medical costs (as shown in **Figure 1**). According to the theory, if the patients have enough knowledge, healthy beliefs, skills, and support, they would try beneficial healthy behaviors. At the same time, the researchers could think from different angles the intervention based on self-management, such as reducing the situation. The risk factors or specific situational factors in environmental factors can strengthen knowledge and belief (such as self-efficacy), enhance individual self-restraint behavior, and increase social support. Therefore, the theory has a profound guiding significance for practice. Now it has been widely used in research design, intervention, and development of measurement tools in self-management behavior research and has been verified in a variety of situations and groups of people [5].

Self-efficacy is the core concept in social cognitive theory, which is usually used to assess the efficiency of self-management in chronic disease such as arthritis, diabetes, heart disease, and so on [6]. Improving the level of self-efficacy, which includes developing related knowledge and skills, as well as confidence in individual's ability to accomplish the task/aim in a specific environment, changes behaviors in pain management. Through personal experiences or from the experiences of others, self-efficacy would be improved [7].

2. Self-efficacy for rheumatoid arthritis

Self-efficacy is an index to assess persons' confidence to perform an appointed task or behavior, which is one of the most important factors in terms of personal behavior. Self-efficacy is the core concept of Bandura's social learning theory that attempted to predict the human behavior by referring to the assessment of an individual's competence towards a specific behavior successfully [8]. The self-efficacy theory suggests that the most influential elements for changing health behaviors are perceived threat (influenced by perceived severity and susceptibility to the disease and cues to action, such as increased disease symptoms and advice from others), perceived barriers to using health behaviors, and self-efficacy which would bring the benefits on health behaviors (outcome expectancy) and person's ability (efficacy expectancy).

Thus, self-efficacy of health behavior confirmed the persons' needs to take appropriate and meaningful action. It is nowadays the important theory in predicting and guiding health behavior. Meanwhile, some studies confirmed that the perceived ability to perform a given behavior is strongly related to one's actual performance of the behavior.

3. Review of self-management interventions in rheumatoid arthritis

A recent meta-analysis revealed that such interventions provide additional benefits for pain relief 20–30% as great as the effects of nonsteroidal anti-inflammatory drug treatments [9].

The researchers suggest that the influence of self-management programs on pain and disability is small yet significant. The researches on self-management program for patients with rheumatoid arthritis have focused primarily on patient education, self-expression, pain management, stress management, and depression management. The arthritis self-management program (ASMP) has been confirmed effective [10]. In general, self-management programs bring many benefits and decrease the medical costs in the long term. Now self-management programs have been recommended by the US National Arthritis Action Plan as an important component of rheumatic care.

4. Traditional patient education

Traditional patient education programs are typically designed to encourage behavioral change and to promote healthy living by lectures or videos. The general intent of patient education programs is to provide information to patients with rheumatoid arthritis regarding ways to modify or adjust essential daily activities to circumvent limitations associated with the disease process [11]. Several studies confirm that support the benefits of educational programs as evidenced by improvements in pain and functional and psychological status; those programs that also incorporated behavioral interventions revealed many good benefits [12].

Traditional patient education is the important part in treatment and nursing. Hence, it would be helpful to enlist advantages and disadvantages for educational relevance. Now the researchers look for better methods on patient education.

5. Mail-delivered, tailored self-management intervention

Mail-delivered, tailored self-management intervention (SMART) is a "tailored print intervention" in which the intervention is tailored specifically to the diagnosis information, medical and nursing problems, physical symptoms,

Number	Content
1	"Self-test" to help people determine how arthritis affects their lives and how to use with the tool kit. The items include pain, fatigue, physical limitations, and health worries
2	Information sheets: working with your doctor and nurse, exercise, medications, healthy eating, fatigue and pain management, finding community resources, and dealing with your emotions
3	Information sheets on key process components of the ASMP: action planning, problem solving, deciding what to try, and individualizing an exercise program
4	*The Arthritis Helpbook*
5	Audio relaxation and exercise compact discs (CDs)
6	Audio CD of all material printed on the information sheets

Table 1.
Mail-delivered, tailored self-management intervention kit.

characteristic of demographics, health status, medications, self-efficacy, and other personal features of the patients with osteoarthritis or rheumatoid arthritis [13]. SMART based on a one-page arthritis questionnaire can construct literally billions of patient-specific responses. The elements include a questionnaire asking questions about pain disability, exercise levels, and other arthritis-related behaviors (**Table 1**) [14]. They are mailed to a central processing center. Each successive letter builds on patient's information from before and rewards positive changes and gives expanded recommendations when appropriate. Each intervention in mailing kits was done 4 months after the results from the previous assessment in patients with rheumatoid arthritis. Hence, the actual length of the intervention ranged from 12 to 18 months. Self-management kits by mail-delivered could be a good alternative for patients who cannot participate in classroom sessions or community lectures, as well as for those in locations and times where there are not enough potential patients to offer classes or lectures. A mailed arthritis self-management tool kit proved effective in improving health status, health behavior, and self-efficacy variables than traditional patient education such as subject talks [15].

Last but not the least, the intervention by mail is a good method of self-management in patients with rheumatoid arthritis. It is more convenient than traditional patient education. But the effect of intervention has been easily influenced by patients' education, age, and other factors. Moreover, it is limited by public services, for example, postal service [16].

6. Internet-based education

Internet-based education provides consistent program delivery, because both the content and process are programmed [17]. The Internet arthritis self-management program consists of password protected, interactive, web-based instruction (The Learning Center); web-based bulletin board discussion (the discussion center); tools that the participants can use individually, such as exercise limbs, medication diaries, and tailored exercise programs (Tools); and *The Arthritis Helpbook*, which contains all of the program content. Meanwhile, it contains discussions of the major types of arthritis and medications and has drawings of suggested exercises [18]. The Internet-based arthritis self-management program (ASMP) proved effective in improving health status in 1 year and is better than the small-group ASMP. In addition, some researches confirm the emerging literature supporting acceptance and utility of Internet-based programming as a venue for self-management education and social support system among individuals with chronic diseases [19].

The results of many researches show that the Internet-based education in arthritis self-management is better than group education or traditional self-management. However, the researchers found that the limitations of Internet-based education are that (1) the effects of intervention have been influenced by educational level of patients, (2) the researches cannot supervise the behaviors of patients, and (3) the patients' learning ability affects the results of treatment and nursing [20].

7. Pain management program

Pain has long been considered a significant source of disability and emotional distress for persons with rheumatoid arthritis. Hence, there is an important index or standard in pharmacological and non-pharmacological interventions to manage the consequences of chronic diseases. In addition, some patients with rheumatoid arthritis pain experience only a minimal response to medical intervention, which may lead to pain inadequately managed [21].

Pain management interventions are focused on minimizing the negative emotional memory of chronic pain through the establishment of effective coping strategies [22]. Coping pain skills are used to increasing the available personal resources for managing pain and improving control ability. Emotional disclosure paradigms is a method by encouraging emotional expression of stressful life events; this method is thought to result in decreased pain [23].

There are some empirically based arthritis-specific online sites focused on arthritis self-management. In randomized controlled trial of adults [24], researchers found improvement in health distress, activity limitation, global health, and self-efficacy. A study of an Internet-based self-management program for patients with arthritis found that people in the experimental condition reported lower pain intensity at posttreatment follow-up compared to people in the attention control condition [25].

The painACTION.com is the Internet web of pain management, which includes many informational lectures designed to enhance both knowledge and patient-provider communication; self-assessments that give chronic pain patients the ability to help determine confidence and awareness about self-efficacy; lessons that deal with specific issues that face chronic pain patients and how to better navigate those hurdles; personal stories that allow for sharing of thoughts, feelings, and solutions from other patients suffering with similar conditions; and tools that can help provide chronic pain persons with skill sets to help navigate their chronic pain experiences and interactions with healthcare providers [26].

Prior to developing the arthritis module for painACTION, the researchers conducted an assessment of the needs in 32 people with arthritis and 12 practitioners to learn what was important to include in an online self-management program. Concept mapping of qualitative data revealed that the information about self-management and chronic pain in the literature and in the other modules on painACTION was desired [27]. When the arthritis module was completed, researchers conducted a randomized controlled trial to assess the efficacy of the program for people with arthritis pain. It was hypothesized that patients randomized to the painACTION intervention would report increased positive cognition, reduced negative cognition, increased frequency of self-management behaviors [28], reduced pain, and improved functioning compared to those in the control condition [29].

Perhaps those with arthritis pain who receive an independent online self-management intervention require more than 6-month period for cognitive changes in self-efficacy and decrease pain level in arthritis. In addition, future researches of online interventions with patients with arthritis could emphasize setting-specific personal health behavior goals that are tracked and monitored over time to help maximize the potential impact on pain [30].

8. Stress management programs

Stress defined as a demand upon an organism to respond to environmental changes may have important implications on the course of rheumatoid arthritis [31]. Psychological responses to stress that might lead to physical function dysregulation can be decreased by interventions aimed at reducing psychological stress. In the research, stress management program usually consisted of four individual 1-hour sessions of stress management with a trained therapist over 2 consecutive weeks and included applied, progressive, cue-controlled, and differential relaxed techniques, such as psychological education, breathing, visualization exercises, and so on [32].

Cognitive-behavioral treatments usually include stress management training, which has been used in several researches with persons with rheumatoid arthritis, and results indicate improvements in psychological variables; moreover, the joint tenderness in patients with arthritis has been decreased in some cases [33]. Some researches studied the long-term effects of stress management training on pain behavior exhibited by people with rheumatoid arthritis [34]. However, the results show that stress management based on cognitive-behavioral principles does not have a significant impact on reducing pain behaviors in persons with RA [35].

9. Joint protection education program (JPEP)

Joint protection (JP) is a self-management method which aims to solve physical symptoms of arthritis by reducing pain, inflammation, joint swelling, and preserving joint integrity. Some researches [36] confirm that the use of an educational-behavioral JP program can increase coping ability among people with rheumatoid arthritis and that it is maintained at 6-month period after education. Much of JP education focuses on teaching the use of different movement patterns to perform activities in daily life. Researches of JP education programs have identified that knowledge of JP methods can be improved, as can ability to show JP skills after education [37].

Barry [38] recommended that a number of criteria are followed when developing joint protection programs: conduct a problem analysis at the beginning of the development; use a correct theoretical model; aim to improve knowledge, behavior, and health status; teach effective self-management skills through strengthening self-efficacy and learning knowledge; and involve significant others and accurately evaluate the program. The education program aimed to enhance the self-management strategy. Joint protection skills would be used to assess the effects of them. Joint protection might bring many benefits in self-management and routine care.

10. Exercise program

Although people with arthritis tend to be less fit than their peers without this condition, studies have demonstrated that persons with arthritis can safely participate in appropriate exercise programs to improve their physical fitness, muscular strength, psychosocial status, and functional status [39]. On the basis of these reports and other research findings, healthcare providers have been advising participation in exercise programs for persons with arthritis [40].

The People with Arthritis Can Exercise (PACE) program is a community-based program developed by the Arthritis Foundation in 1987 (revised in 1999) to improve the self-management of arthritis through exercise [41]. This is an 8-week program, administered twice weekly for 1 hour, is offered at disease-management levels, and is available for widespread use in community-based settings [42]. In summary, the study demonstrated that PACE improve symptoms and strength, exercise endurance, and physical activity by offer two times per week. The program was well received by the people with arthritis and instructors in a variety of communities [43].

11. Fatigue management program

Many studies show that fatigue is a major issue, as important as pain, overwhelming, unmanageable, and ignored by clinicians and healthcare providers. The study team developed the cognitive behavior theory (CBT) intervention from chronic pain and fatigue syndrome in arthritis self-management programs, incorporating experiences of rheumatoid arthritis fatigue from clinics, patients, and healthcare providers. The program was piloted, refined, and then co-delivered by clinical psychologist, doctors, nurses, and specialist occupational therapist, with 6 × 2 hour sessions (weeks 1–6), with a 1-hour consolidation session (weeks 7–14) [44]. Thoughts, feelings, and behaviors related to fatigue were addressed using reflective questioning and guided discovery to enable people to work out links by themselves. Problem solving, goal-setting, self-monitoring in activity/rest, and energy management aimed to help people turn cognitive and behavioral changes into improved well-being. CBT for fatigue self-management in rheumatoid arthritis improves fatigue impact, coping and perceived severity, and well-being [45].

12. Self-management program

Self-management is increasingly being accepted as an important part in the management of chronic disease such as hypertension, diabetes, and so on. Self-management interventions (SMI) are patient-centered, problem-focused, and action-oriented, addressing physical and psychosocial issues [46]. It makes use of educational, behavioral, and cognitive strategies to enhance patients' abilities on self-management [47].

Social and economic benefits research on rheumatoid arthritis has related the financial burdens associated with prolonged disability. In response to the need for inexpensive and effective treatments, the utility of the ASMP was confirmed in a number of studies [48]. The arthritis self-management program (ASMP) was designed by the Stanford Arthritis Center and is a community-based patient education program. This program was developed as a result of a measurement of the needs of people with rheumatoid arthritis; the ASMP covers the characteristic of arthritis, conventional uses of medication, exercise, relaxation techniques, joint protection, nutrition, communication with physicians, and evaluation of nontraditional treatments [49]. The ASMP was found to lead to an increase in rheumatoid arthritis knowledge and the adoption of taught behaviors. Participants in the program also decreased pain; the beneficial effects remained at a 20-month follow-up [50].

The ASMP is one of the leading arthritis patient education programs in the world serving thousands of persons with rheumatoid arthritis each year. The program has been modified in recent years. This modification has resulted in improvement use in assessment of arthritis knowledge and has encouraged people with rheumatoid arthritis to seek other Arthritis Foundation services. Meanwhile, the community-based self-management education interventions and the disease-specific Arthritis Self-Help Course (ASHC) have been found to be effective in improving quality of daily life and reducing healthcare costs [51].

RA-SMI has been demonstrated to have many significant benefits. Any contact with healthcare providers with a specific disease focus appears to be beneficial for patients with rheumatoid arthritis. There appear to be additional benefits of adding health professional intervention and SMI. Improvements on depression and mental health were observed in response to the SMI. Moreover, the results were maintained more than 12 months. The study reported that increasing in prescription of DMARDS by patients' medical practitioner should be viewed as a positive and essential strategy for disease modification and reducing impairment and disability. Empowering patients through education may allow them to be more proactive in seeking better evidence-based medical treatments earlier. As it is one of the important studies on RA-SMI future development which is necessary to continue to optimist the positive outcomes of the program. In particular refinement of the program focusing on the SE and pain outcomes needs to be planned, implemented, and evaluated [52].

13. Nurse-led program on RA

Nurses use a booklet of the systematic identification and assess the comorbidities associated with rheumatoid arthritis. In case of a detected risk factor such as hypertension and/or a nonoptimally managed comorbidity such as the lack of vaccination against pneumococcus, the nurse reminds the patient to pay attention to the management of such comorbidity and advises the patient to visit general practitioner or rheumatologist to deal with it. Meanwhile, a report of this visit was sent to the general practitioner and the rheumatologist of each evaluated patient [53].

Palmer et al. demonstrate [54] the short-term benefit of a nurse-led program on RA comorbidity management and the impact of patient self-assessment of disease activity on rheumatoid arthritis treatment intensification. Nurse-led programs have demonstrated their benefit in the cost-effective management of disease risk factors and improved pneumococcal vaccination coverage in at-risk patients and the management of osteoporosis with fracture risk in older women. Such evidence is not yet achieved in the field of rheumatoid arthritis [55, 56].

14. Critical assessment of self-management approaches

Outcome research on the effectiveness of self-management programs for people with rheumatoid arthritis is encouraging. However, support systems for the efficacy of some interventions have been confounded by methodological limitations. For example, the small sample sizes found in many researches have limited the conclusiveness of the results. Additional missing rates are a major obstacle when studying chronic disease and are especially problematic in the context of rheumatoid arthritis due to the associated physical discomfort and disability. Such factors, in addition to the diagnostic ambiguity of early-stage rheumatoid arthritis, pose methodological challenges. In summary, randomized trials and longitudinal designs have produced the most definitive results regarding the utility of self-management in rheumatoid arthritis [57].

Self-management programs that focus on active coping, such as cognitive restructuring and relaxation training, appear to be more helpful than passive approaches that do not encourage the application of learned skills. Overall, the preponderance of evidence suggests that self-management programs for rheumatoid arthritis are generally helpful for reducing the emotional responses commonly associated with the disease. Clearly, reductions in pain and disability can lead to improved quality of daily life; self-management programs also appear to help offset the cumulative direct and indirect costs associated with rheumatoid arthritis [58].

15. Practical implications for self-management methods

The success of self-management programs for rheumatoid arthritis is based on several factors. First of all, specific skills set for the facilitator and participant are required for different programs. For instance, programs focused on stress and depression management frequently involve strategies which require facilitators to have adequate training in cognitive-behavioral interventions [59]. Additionally success is contingent upon participants motivation and ability to implement learned strategies in their daily life [60].

Secondly, adequate financial resources are often required for many programs; self-management programs typically require nominal yet potentially significant, fees for materials such as workbooks and instructor costs. Given that rheumatoid arthritis can lead to sizeable economic demands as a result of direct and indirect medical costs, additional treatment fees may not be feasible for some persons. Therefore, cost-effectiveness is an important consideration for program development [61].

Last but not the least, physical limitations have been found to impact participant performance and program adherence in programs that employ measures requiring sustained effort or a high degree of geographic mobility [62].

16. Future directions for research and practice

Physical disability and mobility limitations can reduce the ability of persons with RA to participate in treatment outcome studies, so future research might examine the development of self-management programs for persons with RA who have severe physical limitations [63]. Specifically, Internet-based delivery systems may help to overcome the major accessibility challenges. From a methodological standpoint, randomized controlled trials have much to offer to the study of self-management interventions. Without randomization, comparison groups can differ on many potentially confounding variables. Similarly, sample sizes must be adequate in order for the literature to evolve in a definitive manner. Non-randomized designs may be useful in some contexts, but randomized trials with a sufficient number of participants will be critically important for future research on the effectiveness of self-management interventions [64].

Studies of self-management programs that include examination of medical cost offset will be highly advantageous. Evaluation of the cost-effectiveness of self-management programs will be particularly crucial for improving access and third-party reimbursement for psychosocial interventions. Longer-term follow-up of these patients will be of interest to evaluate the sustainability of the observed results, in particular with regard to the management of comorbidities but also in checking the potential impact of the disease activity self-assessment program on other outcomes such as disease activity and/or functional impairment [65].

Meanwhile, the study found that brain biomarkers of how people deal with health information may be one of the important characteristics on which to individualize health education to optimize self-management in disease [66]. The use of brain biomarkers will facilitate the generalizability and reproducibility of research findings and benefit self-management [67]. It is an important research direction in the future.

Author details

Wen Luo*, Xiuli Zhang and Kaijing Ren
Tianjin Hospital, Tianjin, China

*Address all correspondence to: wl1984@yahoo.com

References

[1] Curtis JR, Arora T, Narongroeknawin P, et al. The delivery of evidence-based preventive care for older Americans with arthritis. Arthritis Research & Therapy. 2010;**12**:R144

[2] Dowman B, Campbell RM, Zgaga L, et al. Estimating the burden of rheumatoid arthritis in Africa: A systematic analysis. Journal of Global Health. 2012;**2**(2):020406

[3] Fontaine KR, Heo M. Changes in the prevalence of US adults with arthritis who meet physical activity recommendations, 2001-2003. Journal of Clinical Rheumatology. 2005;**11**:13-16

[4] Lethbridge-Cejku M, Schiller JS, Bernadel L. Summary health statistics for US adults: National Health Interview Survey, 2002. Vital Health Statistics 10. 2004;**222**:1-151

[5] Ryan P, Sawin KJ. The individual and family self-management theory: Background and perspectives on context, process, and outcomes. Nursing Outlook. 2009;**57**(4):217-225

[6] Bandura A. Self-efficacy: Towards a unifying theory of behavioural change. Psychological Review. 1977;**84**:191-215

[7] Hammond A. Adherence with joint protection education. JNAROT. 1997;**11**:84-87

[8] Hewlett S, Carr M, Ryan S, et al. Outcomes generated by patients with rheumatoid arthritis: How important are they? Musculoskeletal Care. 2005;**3**:131-142

[9] Superio-Cabuslay E, Ward MM, Lorig K. Patient education interventions in osteoarthritis and rheumatoid arthritis: A meta-analysis comparison with non-steroidal anti-inflammatory drug treatment. Arthritis Care and Research. 1996;**9**:292-301

[10] Strand V, Singh JA. Improved health-related quality of life with effective disease-modifying antirheumatic drugs: Evidence from randomized controlled trials. The American Journal of Managed Care. 2007;**13**(Suppl 9):S237-S251

[11] Rippey RM, Bill D, Abeles M, et al. Computer-based patient education for older persons with osteoarthritis. Arthritis and Rheumatism. 1987;**30**:932-935

[12] Suurmeijer TP, Waltz M, Moum T, et al. Quality of life profiles in the first years of rheumatoid arthritis: Results from the EURIDISS longitudinal study. Arthritis and Rheumatism. 2001;**45**:111-121

[13] Gale F, Kirk J, Davis R. Patient education and self-management: Randomized study of effects on health status of a mail-delivered program. Arthritis and Rheumatism. 1994;**37**:S197

[14] Goeppinger J, Lorig KR, Ritter PL, et al. Mail-delivered arthritis self-management tool kit: A randomized trial and longitudinal followup. Arthritis & Rheumatism (Arthritis Care & Research). 2009;**61**(7):867-875

[15] Lorig KR, Ritter PL, Laurent DD, et al. Long-term randomized controlled trials of tailored-print and small-group arthritis self-management interventions. Medical Care. 2004;**42**:346-354

[16] Fries J, Carey C, McShane D. Patient education in arthritis: Randomized controlled trial of a mail-delivered program. The Journal of Rheumatology. 1997;**24**:1375-1383

[17] Trudeau KJ, Pujol L, DasMahapatra P, Wall R, Black RA, Zacharoff K. A randomized controlled trial of an online self-management program for adults with arthritis

pain. Journal of Behavioral Medicine. 2015;**38**(3):483-496

[18] Shigaki CL, Smarr KL, Siva C, et al. RA-Help: An online intervention for individuals with rheumatoid arthritis. Arthritis Care & Research (Hoboken). 2013;**65**(10):1573-1581

[19] Shigaki CL, Smarr KL, Gong Y, Donovan-Hanson K, Siva C, Johnson RA, et al. Social interactions in an online self-management program for rheumatoid arthritis. Chronic Illness. 2008;**4**:239-246

[20] Kind T, Huang ZJ, Farr D, et al. Internet and computer access and use for health information in an under-served community. Ambulatory Pediatrics. 2005;**5**(2):117-121

[21] Jenkinson CM, Doherty M, Avery AJ, et al. Effects of dietary intervention and quadriceps strengthening exercises on pain and function in overweight people with knee pain: A randomized controlled trial. BMJ. 2009;**339**:b3170

[22] Multon KD, Parker JC, Smarr KL, Stucky RC, Petroski G, Hewett JE, et al. Effects of stress management on pain behavior in rheumatoid arthritis. Arthritis Care and Research. 2001;**45**:122-128

[23] Keefe FJ, Van Horn Y. Cognitive-behavioral treatment of rheumatoid arthritis pain: Maintaining treatment gains. Arthritis Care and Research. 1993;**6**:213-222

[24] Brosseau L, Wells GA, Brooks S, et al. People getting a grip on arthritis II: An innovative strategy to implement clinical practice guidelines for rheumatoid arthritis and osteoarthritis patients through Facebook. Health Education Journal. 2013;**73**(1):109-125

[25] Somers TJ, Keefe FJ, Carson JW, et al. Pain catastrophizing in borderline morbidly obese and morbidly obese individuals with osteoarthritic knee pain. Pain Research & Management. 2008;**13**:401-406

[26] Newman S, Steed L, Mulligan K. Self-management interventions for chronic illness. Lancet. 2004;**364**(9444):1523-1537

[27] Vironique Vermaak N, Briffa K, Langlands B, et al. Evaluation of a disease specific rheumatoid arthritis self-management education program, a single group repeated measures study. BMC Musculoskeletal Disorders. 2015;**16**:214

[28] Taal E, Rasker JJ, Wiegman O. Patient education and self-management in the rheumatic diseases: A self-efficacy approach. Arthritis Care and Research. 1996;**9**(3):229-238

[29] Romano JM, Jensen MP, Turner JA. The chronic pain coping inventory-42: Reliability and validity. Pain. 2003;**104**:65-73

[30] Bradley LA, Young LD, Anderson KO, et al. Effects of psychological therapy on pain behavior of rheumatoid arthritis patients: Treatment outcome and six-month followup. Arthritis and Rheumatism. 1987;**30**:1105-1114

[31] de Brouwer SJ, Kraaimaat FW, Sweep FC, et al. Experimental stress in inflammatory rheumatic diseases: A review of psychophysiological stress responses. Arthritis Research & Therapy. 2010;**12**:R89

[32] Shearn MA, Fireman BH. Stress management and mutual support groups in rheumatoid arthritis. The American Journal of Medicine. 1985;**78**:771-775

[33] Anderson KO, Keefe FJ, Bradley LA, et al. Predictions of pain behavior and functional status of rheumatoid

arthritis patients using medical status and psychological variables. Pain. 1988;**33**:25-32

[34] de Brouwer SJM, van Middendorp H, Kraaimaat FW, et al. Immune responses to stress after stress management training in patients with rheumatoid arthritis. Arthritis Research & Therapy. 2013;**15**:R200

[35] Parker JC, Smarr KL, Buckelew SP, et al. Effects of stress management on clinical outcomes in rheumatoid arthritis. Arthritis and Rheumatism. 1995;**38**:1807-1818

[36] Brattstrom M. Joint Protection—Rehabilitation in Chronic Rheumatic Disorders. 2nd ed. London: Wolfe Medical Publications; 1987

[37] Hammond A, Lincoln N, Sutcliffe L. A crossover trial evaluating an educational-behavioral joint protection programme for people with rheumatoid arthritis. Patient Education and Counseling. 1999;**37**:19-32

[38] Barry MA, Purser J, Hazleman R, et al. Effect of energy conservation and joint protection education in rheumatoid arthritis. British Journal of Rheumatology. 1994;**33**:1171-1174

[39] Callahan LF, Mielenz T, Ferburger J, et al. A randomized controlled trial of the people with arthritis can exercise program: Symptoms, function, physical activity, and psychosocial outcomes. Arthritis and Rheumatism. 2008;**59**(1):92-101

[40] Minor MA, Hewett JE, Webel RR. Efficacy of physical conditioning exercise in patients with rheumatoid arthritis and osteoarthritis. The Journal of Rheumatology. 1989;**15**:905-911

[41] Mendelson AD, McCullough C, Chan A. Integrating self-management and exercise for people living with arthritis. Health Education Research. 2011;**26**(1):167-177

[42] Minor MA. Exercise and physical activity conference, St. Louis, Missouri: Exercise and arthritis "we know a little bit about a lot of things..." [editorial]. Arthritis and Rheumatism. 2002;**2003**(49):1-2

[43] Brorsson S, Hilliges M, Sollerman C, et al. A six-week hand exercise programme improves strength and hand function in patients with rheumatoid arthritis. Journal of Rehabilitation Medicine. 2009;**41**:338-342

[44] Hewlett S, Ambler N, Almeida C, et al. Self-management of fatigue in rheumatoid arthritis: A randomised controlled trial of group cognitive-behavioural therapy. Annals of the Rheumatic Diseases. 2011;**70**:1060-1067

[45] Kirwan JR, Minnock P, Adebajo A, et al. Patient perspective: Fatigue as a recommended patient centered outcome measure in rheumatoid arthritis. The Journal of Rheumatology. 2007;**34**:1174-1177

[46] Lorig KR, Ritter P, Stewart AL, et al. Chronic disease self-management program: 2-year health status and health care utilization outcomes. Medical Care. 2001;**39**:1217-1223

[47] Arthritis Foundation, Association of State and Territorial Health Officials, Centers for Disease Control and Prevention. National Arthritis Action Plan: A Public Health Strategy. Arthritis Foundation: Atlanta; 1999

[48] Lorig KR, Holman H. Self-management education: History, definition, outcomes, and mechanisms. Annals of Behavioral Medicine. 2003;**26**(1):1-7

[49] Lorig KR, Ritter PL, Laurent DD, et al. The Internet-based arthritis self-management program: A one-year

randomized trial for patients with arthritis orfibromyalgia. Arthritis and Rheumatism. 2008;**59**(7):1009-1017

[50] Fries JF, Spitz P, Kraines RG, et al. Measurement of patient outcomes in arthritis. Arthritis and Rheumatism. 1980;**23**:137-145

[51] Lorig KR, Mazonson PD, Holman HR. Evidence suggesting that health education for self-management in patients with chronic arthritis has sustained health benefits while reducing health care costs. Arthritis and Rheumatism. 1993;**36**:439-446

[52] Lorig K, Ritter PL, Plant K. A disease-specific self-help program compared with a generalized chronic disease self-help program for arthritis patients. Arthritis and Rheumatism. 2005;**53**:950-957

[53] Dougados M, Soubrier M, Perrodeau E, et al. Impact of a nurse-led programme on comorbidity management and impact of a patient self-assessment of disease activity on the management of rheumatoid arthritis: Results of a prospective, multicentre, randomised, controlled trial (COMEDRA). Annals of the Rheumatic Diseases. 2015;**74**:1725-1733

[54] Palmer D, El Miedany Y. From guidelines to clinical practice: Cardiovascular risk management in inflammatory arthritis patients. British Journal of Community Nursing. 2013;**18**:424-428

[55] Koksvik HS, Hagen KB, Rodevand E, et al. Patient satisfaction with nursing consultations in a rheumatology outpatient clinic: A 21-month randomized controlled trial in patients with inflammatory arthritis. Annals of the Rheumatic Diseases. 2013;**72**:836-843

[56] Ndosi M, Lewis M, Hale C, et al. The outcome and cost-effectiveness of nurse-led care in people with rheumatoid arthritis : A multicentre randomised controlled trial. Annals of the Rheumatic Diseases. 2014;**73**:1975-1982

[57] Gallant MP. The influence of social support on chronic illness self-management: A review and directions for research. Health Education & Behavior. 2003;**30**:170-195

[58] de Jong Z, van der Heijde D, McKenna SP, et al. The reliability and construct validity of the RAQoL: A rheumatoid arthritis-specific quality of life instrument. British Journal of Rheumatology. 1997;**36**:878-883

[59] Jorge MT, Jean YR, Mare CH. Rheumatic and musculoskeletal disease and impaired quality of life: A challenge for rheumatologists. Journal of Rheumatology. 1996;**23**:1-3

[60] Riemsma RP, Taal E, Rasker JJ. Group education for patients with rheumatoid arthritis and their partners. Arthritis and Rheumatism. 2003;**49**:556-566

[61] Jordan KP, Joud A, Bergknut C, et al. International comparisons of the consultation prevalence of musculoskeletal conditions using population-based health care data from England and Sweden. Annals of the Rheumatic Diseases. 2013;**73**:212-218

[62] Fontaine KR, Bartlett SJ, Heo M. Are health care professionals advising adults with arthritis to become more physically active? Arthritis and Rheumatism. 2005;**53**:279-283

[63] Iversen MD, Hammond A, Betteridge N. Self-management of rheumatic diseases: State of the art and future perspectives. Annals of the Rheumatic Diseases. 2010;**69**(6):955-963

[64] Parker JC, Smarr KL, Buckelew SP, et al. Effects of stress management

on clinical outcomes in rheumatoid arthritis. Arthritis and Rheumatism. 1995;**38**:1807-1818

[65] Cross MJ, March LM, Lapsley HM, et al. Patient self-efficacy and health locus of control: Relationships with health status and arthritis-related expenditure. Rheumatology (Oxford). 2006;**45**:92-96

[66] Shirley MM, Carol MM, Anthony IJ, et al. Characterization of brain signatures to add precision to self-management health information interventions. Nursing Research. 2019; **68**(2):127-134

[67] Gayle GP, Elizabeth JC, Susan GD, et al. Biomarkers as common data elements for symptom and self-Management science. Journal of Nursing Scholarship. 2018;**50**(3):276-286